Healthy Black Life
A Cultural Guide to Better Health

Paula Watson Gardner

SQUARE TREE PUBLISHING

www.SquareTreePublishing.com

Advice and information contained in this book are for your general guidance only and should not be used in the place of qualified medical advice. The author and publisher cannot take responsibility for any injury sustained as a result of activities and exercises described in this book. Please ensure that you consult your General Practitioner before engaging in exercise or a fitness regime.

For more information about bulk purchases, please contact Square Tree Publishing at info@squaretreepublishing.com.

Cover design by Sharon Marta
Illustrations from Vectorstock

ISBN 978-1-957293-01-1

Table of Contents

—◆●◆—

Introduction

Are you over the age of 35 and sick and tired of feeling sick and tired? If so, then my hope is that this book and the resources available to you will catapult you into a new level of improved health and well-being.

The modern way of life is a result of the many diverse cultures that have been weaved into the fabric of many nations over the years, including Britain, where I currently reside. But with the numerous positives these cultures bring, they bring many challenges as well, especially in the way of health and diet. The Caribbean and African communities add a diverse energy, a platform of faith and a vibrant and flamboyant culture to any society—which is visible across the globe—but what on earth is happening with our health in the process? Why do we find good health and well-being such a challenge today? It seems our moistened skin helps us to look young--we are gifted, and we are black--but we are generally not so healthy.

During the 2020 worldwide Covid-19 pandemic, I was shocked to hear reports in the media that the black community was being adversely affected by this virus, here in the UK, resulting in a high proportion being admitted to Hospital Intensive Care Units (ICU). This, understandably, induced a rippling of fear within our community and questions on why this was the case. The continued reports motivated me to research why, and what, these actual 'underlying issues' happen to be, as there was no mention of specifics in the media. So, this began my in-depth journey of discovery and an ever-increasing desire to learn more about the health of African and Caribbean people across the globe and help find a solution to our poor health.

Working within the health and fitness industry over the past ten years and spending my youthful years as a serious athlete, my heart, skills, and talent lie in the wonders of the human body and how we look after it. I endeavour to help people value and appreciate their body and to make step-by-step improvements that will bring about a more positive health experience in day-to-day living. However, not everyone wants a personal trainer (or can afford one), and not everyone wants to, nor can, rock up to the gym three times a week. This book is primarily for those who would prefer to make lifestyle changes, including dietary adjustments, in their own space or familiar surroundings with friends and family without compromising culture. Because starting a new health regime

Because starting a new health regime can be daunting for some, staying close to home can help you start and continue on your way to a healthy black life.

Healthy Black Life

can be daunting for some, staying close to home can help you start and continue on your way to a healthy black life.

Some of you reading this will be in good health and living your best life; however you may have family members and friends who need encouragement to make a few lifestyle changes. You may have already made a commitment to improving your health and are well on your way to reaching your goals. As you read on, I pray you stay committed to improving your health and encourage you to support your family and friends who decide to take control of their well-being too. Let's be real, some of us would love to see our parents' health improve, right? Becoming a health ambassador to your nearest and dearest has the potential to have a positive impact on family, your social group, and the wider black community, which in turn can start to tilt the scales towards improved health statistics nationally and around the globe. This book will equip you with the information needed to get you, your family, and your friends started on positive change.

This book will equip you with the information needed to get you, your family, and your friends started on positive change.

We will start by looking at our culture, lifestyle, and traditions in order to help pinpoint how we have arrived at where we are on life's health journey, then look ahead to the necessary steps to live a Healthy Black Life.

Acknowledgments

Firstly, I'd like to thank God for giving me the confidence and courage to share my knowledge and for giving me a zeal and passion for life. So much so, that I desire to see others living their best life also.

I would like to thank my gorgeous husband for giving me the space and time to create and write this book. His continued support and encouragement is a true blessing to me, accompanied by his cultural nutritional input as the incredible chef that he is, having spent time living and working throughout West Africa.

I would like to say a big thank you to my family who are a constant joy to my life. My legend of a mother who gave me physical life and has supported me always, I can't thank her enough. My brothers and their families who are such innovators, and a very special mention to my big sis who is always there for me and is such a strong go-getter in life. And last and certainly not least, my beautiful daughter Isla, who is an amazing young woman who continues to inspire me to look up, reach within, and step out. Her awesome achievements thus far have propelled her into a level of success that I admire and am so proud of.

My deepest love to you all!

Paula x

Chapter One

—◆◆◆—

Why Are We So Sick?

The health of the African and Caribbean black community has been challenging in the twenty first century across the western world and continues to flag up issues in today's society. Therefore, there is an urgent need for us to take stock of our lives, recognise issues, and choose to make some simple changes to improve our physical and mental well-being in a world that is unconsciously leading us in the opposite direction. No matter where you are across the globe reading this book right now, Britain, the USA, a Caribbean Island, or the continent of Africa, a few lifestyle and dietary changes can go a long way in making life better for you, your children, and your children's children. After all, we all desire a healthy black life, don't we?

During the past ten years, I have worked within the health and fitness industry and supported many individuals of all backgrounds and cultures who decided to get serious and make the choice to improve their fitness and health. However, over the years, health statistics within the black community have not improved and reports summarise our health as remaining 'poor.' The Covid-19 pandemic raised questions about the unknown reason why a high number of black people were becoming seriously ill. Whilst there are no hard and fast answers to this question, (aside from work, environment, and income), medical professionals do suggest lifestyle and diet as a major factor. This, I'm sure, is the same with all communities, however, the statistics show that there is more of a significant risk for us.

There is a plethora of diet and fitness information on the market today, through books, magazines, social media, and wellness clubs; however, many are generic and have a sense of 'one size fits all' commonality. Very few take into account ethnicity, culture, and tradition regarding food and lifestyle. Our relationship with food and the cultural mindsets we adopt through our parents and upbringing, as well as our environment, builds the foundation of how we think, what we eat, and how we live out our day-to-day lives. I hope this book will reveal some black cultural ideologies that you can relate to in order to identify a pattern in your own life choices that may have contributed to any health concerns.

I am an advocate for helping people live life to the fullest by paying attention to their physical and mental health. Now that I have rolled into my 50s and experiencing crazy changes in my own body, I really would like to reach out to others who want to make changes that will result in more energy, an increased zest for life, a bounce in their step and a new and improved you.

Healthy Black Life

It is clear that the way we live culturally can reveal the good, bad, and the downright ugly habits in our lives. If we are to make successful changes concerning our health, looking back through our cultural eyes may give us insight into habits we have adopted that brought us to where we are today.

Improving your health physically and mentally, and if need be, losing weight, can be easy for some but difficult for others. To be honest, it can be difficult for many of us, especially if we have adopted bad eating and drinking habits as well as a lack of physical exercise. The key is to take it slow, one step at a time, and give yourself the time and space to adjust to new habits. As a society, we put so much pressure on ourselves to change at a fast pace or promote shortcuts to get where we want to be. This is possibly the result of the times we are living in, a type of microwave society where we want things *now*. The so-called advancement of technology to increase speed such as the internet, robotic production lines, online shopping, and even paying your restaurant bill via a mobile app are a handful of ways we are able to save time. Society is encouraging us to develop impatient attitudes and seek instant gratification in life, and this is especially evident in the world of cosmetic surgery, which has accelerated at an incredible rate over the past two decades around the globe. However, faster is not always better in life—just look around at nature; time is an important part of developing beauty in a flower, an

It is clear that the way we live culturally can reveal the good, bad, and the downright ugly habits in our lives.

It's important for us all to remember that time always catches up with us as our tomorrows are the total sum of our todays.

emerging butterfly from its cocoon, or the different seasons that sustain all life. Quicker or easier alternatives can lead to problems down the road, even if at the present time everything looks great. Many people are choosing the easier options in life, after all, the easy way is being offered to us on a plate. However, I believe that this can damage human resilience (strength), which is important to living life. It takes times to develop mental strength, and we all need this to navigate life—especially in difficult times. It's important for us all to remember that time always catches up with us as our tomorrows are the total sum of our todays.

Despite growing older, let's be honest, most of our health concerns are brought on by the following:

- What goes into our bodies (food, drink, substances, the air we breathe, etc.)
- What we choose to give our attention to and feed on mentally (mental health)
- Failing to value the necessity for continued physically activity

Healthy Black Life

My father (of Bajan descent) died at the age of 53 (over 30 years ago) of heart disease following a triple bypass operation he had ten years previously. He had been a smoker for years and spent most of his working day sitting in an office as a manager. I was not close to my father; he left the family home when I was around thirteen years old, but I can honestly say I never saw him exercise or even move at a fast pace, not even a gentle five second jog. Instead, after he arrived home from work, he would consume a small mountain of cultural Caribbean food, leaving nothing except a few gravy lines on his plate.

The combination of all these things had a negative impact on his health. He remarried years after his surgery, and I suspect his diet and lack of exercise did not change. This, coupled with his previous blocked arteries, contributed to his ultimate demise at a relatively young age.

Your personal relationship with food, among other things, can be the reason that led you to where you are today, driven by your mindset and character. However, it is important to mention there could be other physiological concerns our body may be dealing with.

Sports England produced a report called Active Lives Adult Survey November 2018/19 regarding the physical activity of adults in the UK.

In the breakdown of physical activity by ethnicity, the black community were the most inactive group, followed by the Asian community, which had similar health concerns (Black community 58%, Asian community excluding Chinese 54%).

Why Are We So Sick?

In the general population in the UK, the report states:

- *Men are less active than women*
- *The unemployed and lower paid are the least active*
- *Those with long term health issues or disabled are least active*

A UK Government Health Report[1] states the following:

- *In the year to November 2020, 62.8% of adults (people aged 18 and over) in England were overweight or obese*
- *67.5% of Black adults were overweight or obese – the highest percentage out of all ethnic groups*
- *White British adults were more likely than average to be overweight or obese (63.7%)*
- *32.2% of adults from the Chinese ethnic group were overweight or obese – the lowest percentage out of all ethnic groups*

Most of us just need a few lifestyle changes...

Being overweight can be the driver for adopting sickness in our bodies. Some of us may be what the guidelines suggest, slightly overweight or too overweight (labelled obese), but wherever you may be in this range, there are simple steps to help improve your health. Most of us just need a few lifestyle changes and in time,

1 https://www.ethnicity-facts-figures.service.gov.uk/health/diet-and-exercise/overweight-adults/latest#by-ethnicity-over-time

Healthy Black Life

we will notice we have more energy and a reduction in disease in the body, feel better, as well as adopt a more positive outlook on life.

Genetics and hereditary health concerns play a part in this, and these are things that we may not be able to change, so it's important to focus on what we have the capacity to change to stay as healthy as possible.

Medicine is a necessary invention that is a vital part of prolonging our lives, and we should be so grateful for the access we have to it in the UK. The NHS is an incredible institution that supports the fabric of our lives, but we must be careful not to think that this free, easily accessible benefit of modern-day medicine takes precedent over taking responsibility for our own bodies. The healthcare service continues to be overrun with patients, and the medical care workers are continually being overworked because the service is so stretched. Our world is getting sicker in every sense of the word, and so are we (humanity, that is), so taking action to prolong our lives and our world is a necessity now more than ever.

So, let's take a look at where we have come from, where we are today, and the steps we can take to 'live long and prosper' (in the words of Mr. Spock) and enjoy the actual process with friends and family so we are still around to watch our grandchildren grow up.

Chapter Two

———◆●◆———

Cultural History and Lifestyle

Our vibrant culture and traditions have been handed down through generations and are made up of our lifestyle, mental attitudes, diet, faith, and environment. To plan where we want to go in life, or even to find out how we reached where we are today, it is necessary to know where we have come from. I want to take a brief look at our culture and how it has shaped our health through the generations. The way of life in years gone by can bring understanding to what has led us to the health crisis we find ourselves in. Moreover, such reflection can help us plan ahead for improving our health for the future.

...reflection can help us plan ahead for improving our health for the future.

Food

Our ancestors in the time of slavery lived in survival mode, and it was common for their diet to consist of discarded food from the homeowners (masters of the house). Along with the food they grew based on the environment, they created dishes that sustained them after working tirelessly on the plantations or attending to house duties. Some of these dishes have stood the test of time and are the foundation of dishes that have been passed down through the generations. Salting meat and fish was common and was a means to preserving food to stop them from spoiling too quickly. Electric refrigeration was not a common household appliance until the late 1900's and is still missing in many homes today, so salting as well as smoking meat and fish are still common place.

Could this process of salting to preserve be what gave us a palate for richer flavours and a love of salt and spices in our cuisine?

Historically, Caribbean food is a mash up of African, Latin American, European, and Asian cuisine, which was brought in when visitors arrived on our sun-kissed Caribbean shores.

Popular cultural foods we know and love include:

- Rice 'n' Peas
- Macaroni Pie
- Fried Plantain
- Chicken (Jerk, Fried, Broasted)
- Snapper Fish
- Ackee and Saltfish
- Curry Goat
- Yam, Cassava, Sweet Potato, Breadfruit
- A Variety of Meat Such as Corned Beef, Pork, Chicken, and Fish

Healthy Black Life

There is an abundance of tropical fruit such as bananas, coconut, mangos, golden apples, star fruit, soursop and more to enjoy and nourish the body.

On the African continent during the colonial period, European visitors exchanged items such as tomatoes and nuts for African produce, which has impacted food all over the world, from Europe to Latin America. There are many spices and vegetables that are indigenous to Africa, but the foundational staple foods that are quite consistent in meals are generally very similar to the Caribbean diet, including chicken, fish, rice, yam and cassava.

Some traditional food and dishes include:

- Jollof Rice,
- Fufu (Cassava & Plantain)
- Red Red
- Banku
- Eba
- Pepper Soup
- Kontomire Stew
- Chicken
- Moi Moi
- Tilapia Fish
- Chin Chin

Similar to the Caribbean Islands, African cuisine also has a variety of luscious fruit such as bananas, pineapple, pawpaw, coconut, and mangos.

Life was far from easy for the Afro-Caribbean community who arrived in Britain back in the Windrush era, accepting the invitation for employment on the London transport system and the newly formed NHS. Housing rent was high and migrant families struggled to live on low income as well as integrate into a white society. This exposed them to a greater variety of food offered from the British staple diet, as there was limited availability of traditional cultural food items. Still today it is not unusual for us to bring some (or maybe more than some) cultural delights back after a trip back home, because we all know food tastes better when it comes from our homeland. Am I right? This scenario reminds me of a TV programme from Australia called Nothing to Declare, which catches people largely of East Asian descent at the airport who are either on holiday or returning home, with a suitcase full of undeclared food at customs. I find it astonishing to see how much they pack in their bags and suitcases, including delicacies such as bugs and insects to eat or for medicinal purposes. I kid you not!

What sweet drinks come to mind from back home for you?

One thing I notice when I'm back in Barbados is how sweet the drinks are, and I don't mean sweet as in good, I mean sweet as in the sugar content. Oh boy, the local non-alcohol bottled drinks can give you such an energy boost, it's crazy! And too much is seriously not good for your health. What sweet drinks come to mind from back home for you? I'm sure you can think of a few, if not many.

Every year in the UK, someone buys me a bottle of Baileys Original either for Christmas or my birthday; years ago it was my favourite tipple, way before all the varieties existed. I still enjoy a glass now and then, but I find it too sweet at times. On every trip to Barbados, the family would start with buying a few duty-free bottles to enjoy on the island or to take as a gift for family members. My sister would make sure she took advantage of the cheaper booze at London Gatwick or Heathrow in addition to more duty-free at Grantley Adams Airport, Bridgetown. During a trip to Ghana before the pandemic, whilst out and about in the city and around the hotel, I was surprised to see so many men drinking Baileys. I was under the impression it was a chick's drink; however, that may just be the drink culture in the UK.

Could the taste for sugary based, common local items from our homelands, such as Condensed Milk, Guinness Punch, and Milo, be the reason why we are attracted to this creamy, sweet, alcoholic beverage called Baileys? Maybe!

As a child growing up in London, Sunday was cultural food day, and the rest of the week was typically English food from the local shops. I can recall our small kitchen was a hive of activity after church on a Sunday morning. A large pot of rice and various pans sizzling with frying meat and fish on the stove with spices, herbs, onion, flour, and root vegetables, including beetroot scattered on the worktop. It was common for me and my siblings to stay out of the kitchen when mum was cooking, or else be burned by spitting fat from the frying pan or our clothes being consumed with the strong smell of dinner that was lingering in the air, not forgetting the lack of visibility in the room due to excessive amounts of steam.

Cultural History and Lifestyle

Today, I still love a Sunday afternoon at my mother's house when the whole family descends for a lovingly prepared, delicious spread of Caribbean cuisine with a bottle of hot pepper sauce always at hand (I'm a bit of a lightweight when it comes to heat, so I leave well alone)! It's very traditional for my mother to cook 'big food' on a Sunday, even if she doesn't know who, or how many, will turn up. If we didn't, she would just dash any leftovers in the freezer and bring them back out the following weekend. Can anyone else relate? My absolute favourite day for a delicious wholesome meal was, and still remains, Sunday.

It's very traditional for my mother to cook 'big food' on a Sunday, even if she doesn't know who, or how many, will turn up.

I can remember canned corned beef was commonplace in our household. This salted and spiced tinned beef could sit on the cupboard shelf for ages and was a part of our staple diet. We had it on crackers, in sandwiches, on rice, mixed with vegetables—every which way—and I can honestly say I enjoyed it. I believe it is still popular today, as it is relatively cheap and can be purchased anywhere in the world. I also remember the unforgettable smell of saltfish in my mother's cupboard. I still get a whiff of it from time to time when she decides to make a batch of fishcakes on a weekend. They taste so good.

In the 1990s, I worked as a Fleet car sales administrator at a car dealership, and every lunchtime I would visit the cleaning team who prepared brand new cars for delivery to our customers. In those days, the car cleaning team was a great bunch of guys from Nigeria who took pride in their work. They were fun to work alongside, laughing and joking over a bowl of traditional food like fufu or soup, which they would take turns bringing in for lunch. I would always rock up to check on the cars at the right time, so I was always offered some traditional splendour to try, which was full of flavour and very filling. Good times!

Could our history of how we cook and what we eat, especially our staple food consisting of carbohydrates, starchy, high sugar-based products and salt-rich items, be contributing to our present health concerns?

Lifestyle

My parents came to Britain from Barbados in the 1960s along with many others who were invited by the British government to find work and help rebuild society after the second World War. Although this was a great opportunity to start a new life and find employment, it was far from easy. My father arrived before my mother and started work on the London Transport Network whilst my mother started working in local factories after she arrived by boat at the docks in Liverpool. My parents had to work just as hard as everyone else to earn a living, so times were tough. Adjusting to life in a foreign country is hard enough but with darker skin, it made it that much more suppressive.

Strength is a good thing; however, if we are not careful, it can also be rooted in stubbornness.

This treatment against people of colour also prevalent across Africa, Europe, and the USA has been evident for generations. But through all of its injustices, has given us the strength like no other to keep on keeping on, enabling us to stand, which has been established through the grounds of our faith. Strength is a good thing; however, if we are not careful, it can also be rooted in stubbornness.

I first heard the term 'Liming' in Barbados whilst on holiday many years ago and is used to describe when people hang out, usually in a public place, with friends. It's not an unusual sight to see locals relaxing with a cold bottle of Banks beer or a Frutee in the heat and strength of the midday sun, which I'm sure is common all over the Caribbean. If you close your eyes and imagine this scenario (unless you are currently reading this book on a sun-kissed island), you will notice a lack of bodily movement. After all, who is inclined to move around when it's hot? It's much better to reduce perspiration—sweating (glowing for us ladies)—by preserving energy and keeping still, am I right? The only time I dare to exercise or go for a run when I'm in Barbs is early morning, around 8 a.m. latest, otherwise it is just too hot and rapidly drains my energy. So, no surprise, there is a lack of urgency and speed of the locals in their day-to-day. Hands up if you notice the massively reduced pace of life when in the Caribbean (or even the motherland) compared to the UK or USA? Apart from the sun, sea, sand, palm trees, and lovely people, this may be another reason tourists flock to the Caribbean, just to slow down.

Our unconscious behaviour can be passed on to family, therefore influencing our children...

So, if our parents and grandparents grew up with this pace of life, could it have become part of their nature to preserve energy and not be inclined to move, contributing to a lack of exercise, even if they have relocated to colder climates? Our unconscious behaviour can be passed on to family, therefore influencing our children, as well as our children's children, developing a generational pattern.

There are many reasons why some of us choose not to

Healthy Black Life

exercise, and some may be rooted in our generational past. However, a lack of education and encouragement on the importance of exercise can also be a factor.

Attitudes Towards Mental Health

In the UK today, mental health is a prominent talking point, and there are many organisations trying to support and raise awareness of the importance of addressing mental illness.

Maybe our history has cultivated a culture of shame regarding mental illness...

Black history suggests that mental health conditions were possibly ignored, and individuals shunned with little or no support from the community. Therefore, the idea of mental illness was perceived as bad, even evil, maybe punishment from the spirit world or the result of devil worship. Maybe our history has cultivated a culture of shame regarding mental illness, so individuals have chosen not to address or admit to having a problem.

Could our historical attitude towards mental illness be keeping us from seeking help, therefore escalating the problem by delaying treatment?

Smoking marijuana, home and abroad, has been a popular pastime too, especially for men, which impacts brain function negatively with regular use.

Could our smoking habit be a major factor regarding the mental health of black men in our society, young and old?

Faith

Christianity and Islam are the largest faith groups within the African and Caribbean diaspora across the world, with both recognising the importance of the mind and body. Black culture and traditions are deeply rooted in religion and play a major role in many of our lives, impacting our choices, therefore lifestyle.

The Old Testament in the Bible is filled with accounts of God challenging the traditions of His people. Through the Scriptures, the Israelites always turned back to what they knew and struggled to trust God, who wanted to reveal His way was more beneficial to them. They were steeped in tradition and struggled with change, which made them shortsighted and disobedient in God's eyes. This is an example of how tradition can hinder a positive move forward.

Black culture and traditions are deeply rooted in religion...

One thing that I have experienced as a Christian is that my understanding of faith has evolved over the years, which thankfully, has enabled me to grow spiritually. The Bible states, we do not have it all together as we only know in part (1 Corinthians 1:9), so we must make room for new levels of understanding, leading to new ways of thinking and behaviour.

In the New Testament, the Apostle Paul gives the analogy that Christianity is illustrated by the image of a human being. Christ's Body is the Church (Christians), which is the

30

vehicle God uses to reveal Himself, through the renewing of our minds, (Christ Jesus, the Head). (Colossians 1:18)

Does the Church, as a body, look healthy?

Is the relationship between Christ and His Body flowing with ease? Or Is faith and works of His Body (Church) suffering dis-ease?

The Church isn't as attractive or healthy as Christ would like it to be to the world, and I see this reflected in our own physical bodies. Faith without works is dead (James 2:26) so believing that God heals us is vital (faith). However, we must do our part to respect and value the body He has given us to live in (works).

Are we praying for healing, and at the same time, still doing the things that have caused us ill health?

Are we praying for healing, and at the same time, still doing the things that have caused us ill health?

Do we still struggle with trusting God, allowing traditions to take precedent over growing in faith, and therefore adopt the very same shortsightedness His people struggled with in the Bible?

From a biblical perspective, it seems culture and tradition can be a trip hazard for the Church. Maybe we need a new outlook on tradition, not to negate it, but to refresh it to bring out the best in us. If we are not careful, tradition can replace vision and keep us looking in the past instead of embracing the future. If there is too much focus on tradition, looking back can blur our sight and cause us to stumble as we move forward because we do not recognise where we are heading.

If we are not careful, tradition can replace vision and keep us looking in the past instead of embracing the future.

Our faith can reveal what we value in life. We must remember that the spiritual realm is recognised through the physical realm. Our bodies are vessels containing who we are, so to remain effective and love others, shouldn't we value our physical body, the very thing our spirits are held within?

Healthy Black Life

Chapter Three

———◆◆———

Health Conditions Among the Black Community

Let's turn our attention to the health conditions that affect the black community. Below are known diseases that are common among us with causes that could be leading us down this unhealthy life journey.

- Hypertension (High Blood Pressure)
- High Cholesterol
- Obesity
- Type II Diabetes
- Cancer
- Mental Health

Do you identify with any of these health concerns?

Let's take a brief look at each one now, then investigate symptoms and prevention, as well as other health concerns later on towards the end of the book.

Hypertension (High Blood Pressure)

High blood pressure (HBP) is a common ailment and simply means that your heart is working overtime to keep your blood pumping around the body because of narrowing of the arteries.

Common causes:

- Eating Too Much Salt
- Lack of Exercise
- Bad Diet (Too Much Sugar, Fats, and Processed Foods)
- Smoking
- Being Overweight

High Cholesterol

Cholesterol is made up of different types of fat and is produced by your liver, however, it is also prevalent in food. If too much is found in our blood, over time it will clog up blood vessels, sticking to the sides, thus restricting blood flow and having the potential to enter major organs.

Common Causes:

- Eating Food with a High Fat Content
- Being Overweight
- Lack of Exercise
- Alcohol
- Smoking

Obesity

The term *obese* is used by medical professionals to indicate that a person's body weight is too high in comparison to their height.

Day-to-day problems related to obesity or being overweight include[1]:

- *Breathlessness*
- *Increased Sweating*
- *Snoring*
- *Difficulty Doing Physical Activity*
- *Often Feeling Very Tired*
- *Joint and Back Pain*
- *Low Confidence and Self-Esteem*

...obese is used by medical professionals to indicate that a person's body weight is too high in comparison to their height.

1 https://www.nhs.uk/conditions/obesity/

Common Causes:

- Too Much Food
- Too Little Movement

If the pancreas cannot produce enough insulin to cope with the high levels of sugar, then sugar stays in the bloodstream...

Type II Diabetes

A major health concern for people who are overweight and have a high waist measurement is the onset of Type II diabetes where the cause is attributed to the surplus of glucose (sugar) in the blood. Insulin is released from the pancreas to breakdown the sugars and remove them from the bloodstream. If the pancreas cannot produce enough insulin to cope with the high levels of sugar, then sugar stays in the bloodstream leading to a number of more serious health concerns.

L.M. Goff's article, Ethnicity and Type II diabetes in the UK, states:

Type 2 diabetes is a major UK public health priority. Among minority ethnic communities, the prevalence is alarmingly high, approximately three to five times higher than in the white British population. Particularly striking is the earlier onset of Type 2 diabetes, which occurs some 10-12 years younger, with a significant proportion of cases being diagnosed before the age of 40 years. This review focuses on the UK context and Type 2 diabetes in adult populations,

Healthy Black Life

exploring the available evidence regarding the complex interplay of biological, lifestyle, social, clinical and healthcare system factors that are known to drive these disparities.[2]

Age, family history, and ethnicity can contribute to someone's risk, with people of African-Caribbean, Black African or South Asian descent two to four times more likely to develop Type 2 diabetes than white people.

...with people of African-Caribbean, Black African or South Asian descent two to four times more likely to develop type 2 diabetes than white people.

The single greatest risk factor, however, is obesity. While not every case of Type 2 diabetes is associated with excessive weight, it is responsible for 80 to 85% of someone's risk of developing the condition.[3]

Common Causes:

- Obesity
- Bad Diet
- Not Enough Movement (Exercise)

---

2 https://pubmed.ncbi.nlm.nih.gov/30614072/

3 https://www.diabetes.org.uk/about_us/news/diabetes-prevalence-2019

Cancer

As we age, the risk of developing cancer increases, and research shows that figures are high among the black community. The more common diagnoses are:

- Breast
- Prostate
- Lung
- Colon/Rectal

Common Causes:

- Smoking
- Alcohol
- Unhealthy Diet
- Obesity
- Old Age

Mental Health

Mental health has a huge impact on our physical body; after all, our mind and body work together to create our life. Whenever you are anxious, fearful, or stressed, a

Healthy Black Life

hormone called cortisol is released into the bloodstream. Too much cortisol in the body on a regular basis can have a detrimental effect and lead to disease. High blood sugar levels (Type II diabetes) can also negatively affect our mental health, creating mood changes which can raise anxiety levels, leading to an onset of depression and fatigue.

BAME (Black, Asian and Minority Ethnic) and Mental Health

There are a number of variables that the ethnic communities encounter which can influence mental health:

High blood sugar levels (Type II Diabetes) can also negatively affect our mental health...

- *Social and Economic*
- *Racism and Discrimination*
- *Mental Health Stigma Among the Communities*
- *Criminal Justice System*

Different communities understand and talk about mental health in different ways. In some communities, mental health problems are rarely spoken about and can be seen in a negative light. This can discourage people within the community from talking about their mental health and may be a barrier to engagement with health services.[4]

The Adult Psychiatric Morbidity Survey (APMS) found that black men were more likely than their white counterparts to experience a psychotic disorder in the last year.

---

4 https://www.mentalhealth.org.uk/

Risk of psychosis in Black Caribbean groups is estimated to be nearly seven times higher than in the White population.

Risk of psychosis in Black Caribbean groups is estimated to be nearly seven times higher than in the White population.

Detention rates under the Mental Health Act during 2017/18 were four times higher for people in the 'Black' or 'Black British' group than those in the 'White' group. Black men were reported to have the highest rates of drug use and drug dependency than other groups.

Whilst the White Caucasian population experienced the highest rates for suicidal thoughts, suicide rates are higher among young men of Black African, Black Caribbean origin, and among middle aged Black African, Black Caribbean and South Asian women than among their White British counterparts.[5]

Summary

So, looking briefly at health within the black community, it's important that we take a good look at where we are and turn back instead of continuing on this road to even poorer health. As you read this book, think about the changes you can make to start your journey to better health, no matter how small. What's important is a commitment to make changes if you want to improve your health and well-being.

---

5 https://www.mentalhealth.org.uk/

Chapter Four

---◆◆◆---

Our Relationship with Food

The number one purpose for the consumption of all food and drink is to keep us ALIVE AND KICKING. Yes, folks, its primary goal is to maintain the status quo and to keep the body working efficiently and effectively. However, because of the abundance of food available to most of us, we could be forgiven for thinking that food and drink only exists to satisfy two senses—hunger and pleasure. Have you heard the phrase, 'You are what you eat?' This is a very true statement because what you choose to put in your body—whether good or bad and the amount—will determine how your body will function.

...what you choose to put in your body—whether good or bad and the amount—will determine how your body will function.

In the UK, the abundance of diverse food and drink in the supermarket is incredible. However, it seems that looks and the taste of our food is prioritized over its ability to provide nourishment and good health. We try to satisfy two of our senses before we even consider the nutritional value and the calorific content of the food we eat.

We live in a consumer age which caters to our emotions through advertising and marketing to compel us to buy products or support a certain brand. We must understand that we make a lot of daily choices based on our emotions, but the problem with this is that our emotions can change from one moment to the next depending on what is happening in our life on any given day.

When it comes to eating too much of the things we shouldn't, how often do we say, 'One more won't hurt.' I have said it countless times, and I'm sure you have, too. We truly like to kid ourselves in believing that we can get away with feeding on whatever and how much of whatever, we want. Take this phrase, for example: 'What you can't see won't hurt you.' This statement seriously trips us up. We cannot see the calories in our food, but they are definitely there, just like we cannot see a harmful coronavirus, but it currently exists.

...we have developed a particular palate that is drawn towards salt infused and starchy food.

Earlier in the book I mentioned that we love our Afro Caribbean rich flavoured food which has been passed down and developed through the generations. Therefore, we have developed a particular palate that is drawn towards salt infused and starchy food. We are also addicted to sugar, and we continue to digest too much of it. Sugar isn't just found in desserts, but also in the processed savoury food in our diet. Did you know that once digested, simple carbohydrates (bread, pasta, rice, potatoes, pastries, and even milk) convert to sugar (glucose) and is stored in our body until it is needed for fuel (energy)? If we do not use this glucose, your liver will store it in your body as fat. So, eating too much of this type of food, without increasing our movement to burn this excess sugar, will increase our body weight and put us at risk of developing health issues mentioned in the previous chapter.

Seedtime and Harvest

Nature spells it out for us plainly! I absolutely adore my garden and find the most amount of joy wandering around it with a hot mug of tea, watching new shoots appear in the springtime or arming myself with my secateurs, clipping and pruning my flowers and plants. When I see new shoots, I know they are the result of previously planted seeds or bulbs that grew after being fed sunlight and water. Seedtime and harvest is a process of life (you reap what you sow) and it is present in our everyday and in all circumstances. It means specific outcomes will depend on what was done beforehand. Our before determines our today, so I planted the seeds, and then ensured they received water and sunlight so they would grow to their full potential, looking stunning in my garden.

In between the words *seedtime* and *harvest* is the word *and,* which represents the process of time.

So, let's now translate this process to our diet:

Seedtime	=	Food and drink we choose to consume, as well as the quantity
And	=	Digestion
Harvest	=	Impact of the digested food and drink in our body

Your harvest will depend on what seeds you sow, good seed or bad (good food or bad). We need to start paying attention to life's processes, as too often we are playing catch up because we are unhappy with the harvest we are reaping (poor health). If we want an orchard of apples, we need to sow apple seeds. If we want tomatoes, we need to sow tomato seeds. Therefore, if we want a healthy long life, we need to make good lifestyle choices. Do you get the picture? We live in harvest every day because we are planting (making choices) every day of our lives. And I'm not just talking about food either, it's in everything we think, say, and do.

Your harvest will depend on what seeds you sow, good seed or bad (good food or bad).

Life is precious and you are precious, so by understanding the process of seedtime and harvest, a process of life, or Newton's Law ('every action has an equal and opposite reaction'), it can help you make better choices and live a better, healthier, happier, and longer life.

What I am writing may be a new concept to you, a new way of thinking about nutrition. It is important that you pause to take it in and ponder your life choices, because understanding this process can significantly change your circumstances for the better.

You are Wonderfully Made

Your body is amazing and complex with your brain taking care of your bodily functions without you consciously thinking about it. To live a good, healthy, long life, all you have to do, for the most part, is give your body what it needs, physically and mentally, yet it seems we find this to be one of the hardest things to do.

Do you live by doing what feels good instead of doing what is best for you?

Do you live by doing what feels good instead of doing what is best for you?

Do you actually know what is best for you?

What we see, hear, smell, taste, and touch drives our behaviour and runs our lives. Your efficient body can flush out harmful toxins that find their way in via food, drink, air particles, and our skin, to keep the status quo (balance) in our body. However, if we continue to put the wrong things in without enough of the right things, our bodies will let us know. Your body will not flow with ease, it will develop dis-ease.

What we feed ourselves is not limited to the food that enters through our mouths, but also includes what we look at and what we hear, which has a direct impact on our mental health. Can you think of a decision you made based on your emotions, then regretted later? Of course, we have all experienced this, but how often do we do it? We can bring trouble upon ourselves if we allow our emotions to dictate our choices day by day in every area of life.

Emotional Eating

Many who want to lose weight try programmes or clubs such as Slimming World or Weight Watchers in the UK. However, when the goal weight is reached, many people, in time, put the weight back on, and may even end up heavier than when they first started. The way we look at food must change. When we are hungry, we can, unfortunately, choose what to eat through the eyes of feelings.

Do you ever ask yourself, 'What does my body need right now?' instead of, 'What do I feel like eating?'

How we feel can determine what and when we fuel our bodies. Our emotions are fickle and can change in an instant, swinging from one end of the spectrum to the other depending on our circumstances.

Healthy Black Life

I was so fortunate to marry my amazing husband on the shores of Barbados in November 2019, just before the Covid-19 pandemic began to rear its ugly head around the globe. A few days before the wedding, I was so excited and anxious that I could hardly eat. I had to force myself, even though I had planned to only eat small portions (wedding dress nerves). It was as if the excitement and adrenaline were my fuel and I didn't need anything else to carry me through to the big day (oh, except plenty of water, the odd rum sour and a few pina coladas).

Can you think of times when you did not want to eat based on your emotions?

On the flip side, when I have too much to do and don't know where to start, or if I am a bit anxious about a decision I have to make, I will often spend time visiting the kitchen, opening the fridge door looking

...I will often spend time visiting the kitchen, opening the fridge door looking for something to put in my mouth.

for something to put in my mouth. I'm not actually hungry; I think it is a way to distract myself from my discomfort by doing something I enjoy, which is munching good food.

When you are having a crappy day, do you find yourself reaching for high calorie processed comfort food, like cake?

Either way, allowing our emotions to steer our eating and drinking can create a chaotic and potentially unhealthy relationship with what we consume.

Our Relationship with Food

I had to make a conscious effort to disconnect my feelings from my diet, and one way of doing this was to view food differently. *I look at my food as fuel for my body for it to function well and stay healthy.* By looking at it this way, I am able to think more about what my body needs rather than what I feel like eating. Don't get me wrong, I can eat unhealthy food like anyone else. However, it's about how often I allow it, that will affect my health in the long term. If I want to stay loving life and feeling vibrant with high levels of energy, then I must make decisions that will create that reality. Moderation is the key.

If I want to stay loving life and feeling vibrant with high levels of energy, then I must make decisions that will create that reality.

Ask yourself the following questions and be completely honest with yourself. This will help you identify some areas where you need to make an adjustment and become more aware of your current dietary habits.

- Do I overfill my plate, or do I leave space?
- Is there anything I am eating too much of which may be detrimental to my health?
- Do I know about the nutrients in the food I am eating?
- Do I use large amounts of oil whilst cooking?
- Do I eat too much sweet food?
- Do I drink at least eight cups of water a day?
- Do I drink more fizzy drinks than water?
- Do I try to manage my weight?

Healthy Black Life

Chapter Five

———— ◆•◆ ————

Cultural Food Guide to Better Health

In this chapter we look at ideas that could help you with your eating habits as well as alternative food items to consider using whilst cooking. We will also investigate the nutritional content of food and the impact it has in your body to reduce sickness and increase your health.

Below are some useful first step tips and suggestions on getting started. Don't think that you must do everything straight away. In fact, it would probably be better to start with just one thing. Once you start feeling comfortable with that change, take another step. It takes time for your body to adjust to changes, even small ones, so be careful not to take on too much too soon. If you do, you might become frustrated and overwhelmed with too much change at one time and then give up trying.

One Step at a Time Eating Tips

Use a Smaller Dinner Plate

This may sound strange, but the size of your plate really does matter. As I mentioned previously, my father's plate was a normal size dinner plate; however, it was piled up with so much food it looked like a mini mountain. The bigger the plate, the more we generally fill it. Isn't it funny that we need to make sure the whole plate is covered with food for us to call it a meal? How many of us, at a buffet, choose everything we like to eat, but if the plate isn't full and we don't like any other choices, we just take more of what we already have to fill out the plate? Whether we are paying for it or not, our unconscious mind is telling us that to feel satisfied with our meal, we need a full plate of food. If this is our thought pattern, we must reduce the size of the plate so there is less room to fill it. Try it!

The bigger the plate, the more we generally fill it.

I often eat from a side plate and if I am still hungry, I have a bit more. I learnt that even having a little more, I was still reducing my food intake, and psychologically, I felt satisfied because I was clearing my plate. You will probably feel you have eaten enough when the plate is empty, too.

If Possible, Don't Keep Too Much Sweet Food and Drink in the House

Culturally, we do like sugar as it can be found in excess in our food and beverages and this could also be quite a tricky one to master if you have a large family. However, the fewer of these products in your home, the more these items will be out of reach. Maybe substitute those items for fruit or a reduced sugar and fat version, but generally, try to keep most of the naughty stuff out of your basket and leave it on the shelf when you are shopping. We often reach for the same products on our weekly or bi-weekly shop, and we know how long it will last until the next visit. For starters, if you usually buy three packets of biscuits or cookies, try buying two packets instead and challenge yourself to make them last longer.

Cupped Palm Size Portions

When portioning food out, use your hand as a palm-sized cup, especially when portioning out carbohydrates, like rice, pasta, or potatoes. This could help you reduce meal sizes by sticking to no more than two palm-sized cups for this type of food. This works well with reducing the size of your plate too, as mentioned earlier.

Drink a Large Glass of Water Before Your Meal

Don't worry, this will not spoil your meal. The reason for this is to make you feel fuller before you eat, helping you reduce your food intake. Try to drink water instead of sugary drinks, as they add more calories to your meal.

Prepare Meals Ahead of Time

Organising your meals can help you eat less and much healthier as well. We are more likely to eat fast or processed food if we have not planned what to eat ahead of time. This does not mean that you must have all the ingredients ready, but that you have decided beforehand, what to eat so you can keep a balance of good nutrition in your diet.

Reduce the Size of White/Beige Food on Your Plate

The white/beige food on our plate is largely starch based carbohydrates consisting of rice, yam, potato, pasta and other flour-based items. Whilst this food does have some nutritional value, reducing your portion will limit how much food is converted to (glucose) sugar in your body. This can help with weight management and help reverse Type II Diabetes.

Try Not to Add too Much Salt When Preparing Meals

Most of our meals already contain far too much salt, especially shop readymade meals. When we are preparing our cultural dishes, we generally add salt, or substitute seasoning and some can contain too much sodium. Salt pulls fluids from your cells to be processed and this can cause immediate water retention and dehydration, making you feel heavier

...we generally add salt, or substitute seasoning and some can contain too much sodium.

after your meal, even if you are not overeating. Try to reduce salty seasoning or try alternatives with less salt. Too much salt in your diet causes high blood pressure (hypertension) and if it is not addressed, over time can lead to more serious health concerns.

Try to Eat Every 2-3 Hours (Healthy Snack)

It's quite common for people to think if they don't eat for hours on end, then they will lose weight. Even though this is true to some extent, our bodies are remarkable at initiating survival coping mechanisms. If we deny ourselves food for four hours or more, our bodies may decide to hang on to the sugar and fat rather than use it freely. Not eating for long periods of time can make you feel lethargic and tired, making you less likely to move or exercise as it slows down your metabolism. This is not ideal, especially if you are sedentary, sitting down most of the day. Having a small, healthy snack between meals tells your body that food is readily available, so that there is enough constant energy to use instead of your body choosing to store it.

Increase Water, Keep Hydrated

It's a fact that many of us do not drink enough water, only reaching for a glass when we feel thirsty, but by this time, usually dehydration has already set in. Did you know that the feeling of thirst and hunger are quite similar, so sometimes we think we are hungry when actually all we need is to drink a long glass of water. Water is necessary for our basic health and a lack of it can cause problems such as water retention and high blood pressure, which can then put you at risk of developing more serious

A lack of fluid in your body can also increase joint pain and muscle ache and leave you feeling very lethargic and tired.

health issues. A lack of fluid in your body can also increase joint pain and muscle ache and leave you feeling very lethargic and tired. Drinking on average 8 full cups a day of water, plus any other hot or cold beverages (not including alcohol), will help keep your fluids at a healthy level, increase energy, and help flush out any toxins in the blood stream passing them out through your waste.

Try Not to Eat Large Meals Later than 8 p.m.

Most people are winding down by around 8 p.m., using less energy for the rest of the day, therefore there is no need to add more calories to your daily intake. During the night when we sleep, the body goes to work maintaining and repairing the body. It helps if your body isn't trying to digest food at the same time. Sleeping is a type of fasting for the body, so let it do its thing, repairing and restoring your body, instead of trying to digest a late-night meal, especially if it is a cultural meal consisting of meat and rice.

Chew Your Food Well Before Swallowing

If you don't chew your food enough before swallowing, it makes every other stage more difficult...

Digestion begins in the mouth, and chewing your food is important for the next stage of digestion. If you don't chew your food enough before swallowing, it makes every other stage more difficult, which may cause heartburn, bloating, indigestion, and stomach aches. Chewing well is very important, especially when you are eating meat, as it is more difficult for the body to digest.

Try Not to Talk Too Much While Eating

Talking while eating will cause you to take in more air when you are chewing, which can affect the digestion process. Chatting with family or friends while having a meal is common place in society, however, be mindful it can cause indigestion, and even cause you to choke if food passes into the windpipe.

Make Time to Eat, Don't Rush

Taking time to sit and eat can be difficult when we have busy lives, but there are benefits. When you relax while you eat, you can chew your food properly, which aids the digestion process. Eating slowly can also make the meal more pleasurable, allowing you to feel satisfied sooner and prevent overeating.

Keep Your Mind on Eating

Many of us, myself included, can allow our minds to drift as we eat by thinking about what we need to do, events of the day, or even through watching TV. When we are not focused on our food and are mentally distracted, we can miss the meal. What I mean is, you can miss the flavours,

We need to adjust our thinking and dis-associate satisfaction with being full.

the textures, and the enjoyment of what you are eating. This can have a psychological impact in our brain, delaying the trigger of satisfaction and making us want more food until that feeling is reached. I have done this a number of times, finished a meal and then realised I didn't even remember eating it, because my mind was elsewhere. Hands up if you have experienced this? I'm quite sure we all have.

Do Not Eat Until You Cannot Fit in Another Mouthful

We shouldn't eat until we are bursting at the seams and full to the brim, because the pressure of so much food will expand the size of our stomach and could cause heartburn and acid reflux. The larger your stomach, the more food you will have to eat to feel satisfied. This is an unhealthy eating habit which is attached to our emotions and psyche because we associate satisfaction with fullness. We should be eating to feel comfortable at the end of the meal, with room to spare, not until we cannot take another mouthful. We need to adjust our thinking and dis-associate satisfaction with being full.

Do Not Lie Down After Eating a Meal

If you feel lethargic after eating a substantial meal, it's probably because your blood has been directed to your stomach to help digest so much food. We have a name for this feeling in Barbados, I won't mention it, but it ends in 'itus! In order to digest your food

We have a name for this feeling in Barbados, I won't mention it, but it ends in 'itus!

well, it is important that you assist your digestive system by sitting upright to allow the food to travel down into your intestines, allowing gravity to assist. If you lie down, this can disrupt the process and you could experience heartburn and acid reflux of the food back into your throat. I'm sure many of us know what this feels like. Give yourself at least an hour or two before lying down.

Create a Shopping List

Know what you want when you go shopping instead of aimlessly strolling down every aisle in the supermarket, letting your feelings do the shopping. Having a list will help you stay on track and not deviate to other foods that look so yummy but are unnecessary for your chosen meals. Just look for the items on your list and step away from the desserts!

Healthy Black Life

Freeze Down Portions

When cooking pots of food, like curry and stews, invest in some containers that will allow you to freeze individual portions for you to access later. These containers are readily available to buy at the supermarket or local food stores. Or you can wash up the containers from your occasional Chinese, Indian, or Caribbean take away and make use of them.

Eating Out

When visiting a restaurant, reduce your courses. For example, choose two courses instead of the regular three on offer. I have noticed if I go out for a meal, I eat so much more than what I would eat at home, which normally consists of one course. We seem to be programmed to eat several courses, probably because that is what is expected and offered as we gaze through a menu of delicious cuisine that tantalises our tastebuds. To be honest, depending on the size of the portions, just one course will suffice at times. It is perfectly fine to reject the dessert menu when it is offered to you. Honestly, it is fine to reject it!

When cooking pots of food, like curry and stews, invest in some containers that will allow you to freeze individual portions for you to access later.

Eat a Colourful Plate

Try to reduce the amount of white/beige starchy food on your plate and replace it with colour. This will generally be from different vegetables, which will increase the nutritional value of your meal, as well as reducing the starchy content.

Remove the Salt (Sodium) from the Dinner Table

The bottom line is that we consume far too much sodium, as stated earlier. If your meal is rich in flavour through the salt seasoning used during cooking, then there

Too much salt causes High Blood Pressure, and this is a serious problem within the black community...

is no need to add more salt at the dinner table. Sometimes, we pick up the saltshaker out of habit, even before we have tasted our food to see if we need to add any more. Too much salt causes High Blood Pressure, and this is a serious problem within the black community—I can't stress this enough.

Spray Oil When Frying instead of Pouring

To reduce the amount of oil in your food whilst frying, use an oil that you spray instead of a pouring container. You can purchase oil in small, ready spray bottles, or you can purchase an empty refillable spray container for your preferred oil. Spray just enough to coat the surface of your non-stick pan. This will help reduce calories and excess fat intake.

Alternative Cooking Options

African and Caribbean traditional dishes bring a sense of home and love for our rich heritage, and that will always be the case, especially when one is living abroad. Eating a cultural meal gives me a sense of connection and belonging and love for Barbados, the people, the Caribbean, and my African heritage.

How we cook our food has a huge impact on our health if our preferences are unhealthy, i.e. too much frying.

Try to reduce calories when preparing meals by trying some of these alternative cooking options.

Reduce	Substitute with
Shallow Saucepan Frying	Griddle Pan Frying (Minimal Oil)
Deep Frying	Roasting
Broasting (Part Frying)	Grilling
	Air Frying (For Crispy Texture)
	Stewing
	Steaming
	En Papillote (Roast in Foil)
	BBQ

Healthier Food Alternatives

When society discusses diet and cleaner eating, there is a wealth of food and recipe books available in the store or online, created by leading chefs and foodies. Whilst this is very helpful to a lot of people, I find that the Black and Asian community do not buy into this. My understanding is that we learn how to cook from our parents, grandparents, aunties, and uncles. There is no such thing as 2 fluid ounces of this or 100ml of that. Instead, we put in a dash of this and a handful of that. Our food isn't scripted, its foundation is spontaneously embedded firmly within our cultural history. The spices, the smells, the textures, and those mouth-watering flavours are weaved in to who we are. That is why if we are to improve our health through our diet, then it is important that we do so within the realm of our cultural food.

There is no such thing as 2 fluid ounces of this or 100ml of that.

This list of food items below is to help you to think about and experiment with using alternatives to create your favourite dishes. You may need to add more variety to ensure you are giving your body what it needs to support good, healthy living. Remember, in all that we eat and drink, moderation is the key.

Remember, in all that we eat and drink, moderation is the key.

MEAT

Reduce	Alternatives
Red Meat	Chicken
Ham	Turkey
Sausages	Liver
Bacon	Guinea Fowl
Corned Beef	Quorn
Hot Dogs	
Beef Jerky	

It is important to note that mass produced meats contain hormones to increase the growth of the animal and can have a negative impact on the human body. The alternative is to purchase more free range or organic meats or reduce your weekly meat intake.

CHICKEN

It is common to seal in the herbs and spices we use when cooking chicken by coating it with a flour-based mix. This increases and seals the flavour in, as well as giving that crispy coating we all love. Use only a light dusting of flour mix and only give the chicken a quick shallow fry before transferring it to the oven to reduce excess oil. Also, drain off excess fat released from the meat during the cooking process.

Use only a light dusting of flour mix and only give the chicken a quick shallow fry...

STEW

Homemade Stew is a favourite at mealtime and is usually accompanied with rice, potato, yam, or other root vegetables. However, stews can be packed with too much fat, fatty cuts of meat, sodium, and too many calories. Be mindful of your stew's contents; reduce the salty seasoning and cut off excess fat on the meat. Adding some green vegetables can provide needed macronutrients and extra goodness to your meal.

RICE/PASTA

Reduce	Alternatives
White Rice	Brown Rice
Pasta	Quinoa
	Bulgar Wheat
	Couscous
	50/50 Rice (Mixed Brown & White Rice)

DAIRY PRODUCTS

Reduce	Alternatives
Full Fat Milk	Semi or Skimmed Milk & Lactose Free
Cream	Coconut or Almond Milk

Healthy Black Life

Condensed Milk	Low Fat Cream
Full Fat Cheese	Reduced Fat Cheese
Yoghurt	Goats Cheese
	Low Fat Yoghurt
	Probiotic Yoghurt to Aid Digestion
Butter	Reduce Fat/Cholesterol Butter
Margarine	Reduce Fat/Cholesterol Margarine
Ghee	Reduce Fat/Cholesterol Ghee

Reduce High Saturated Hard Cheese	Alternatives
Cheddar	Reduced Fat Hard Cheese
Double Gloucester	Parmesan (Strong, so little is needed)
Blue (Stilton)	Gouda
Swiss	

Reduce Soft Cheeses	Alternatives
Cream Cheese	Feta
Processed Cheese Slices	Mozzarella
	Cottage
	Ricotta
	Camembert

COOKING EGGS

Reduce	Healthier Options
Scrambled	Boiled
Fried	Poached

FATS & OIL

Reduce	Alternatives
Palm Oil (Red Oil)	Olive Oil
Cooking/Saturated Oil	Coconut Oil
	Avocado Oil

It is important to reduce the amount of oil, as much as possible, whilst cooking. How much and what type of oil you use has a huge impact on the calorie content of your meal, therefore your health.

POTATOES

Reduce	Alternatives
White Potato	Red Potato
Yam	Cassava (Yuca Root)
	Sweet Potato
	Bread Fruit

Healthy Black Life

Even though potatoes do have nutritional value, it is important to reduce your portion to one or two cupped palm sizes in your meal to help weight management. If you like chips, air frying and oven baking is a healthier option.

BREAD

Reduce	Alternatives
White/Sugar Bread	Wholemeal Flat Breads/Roti
Hard Dough Breads	Wholegrain & Wholemeal Bread
White Crackers	Wholemeal Flatbread
	Wholemeal Pitta
	Half & Half
	High Fibre Thin Crackers with Reduced Salt

Caribbean and African bread can contain high amounts of sugar with a hard dough consistency. If you make your own, try to reduce the amount of sugar you use.

Try and stick to thin and medium cut slices of bread and reduce how many slices you eat daily.

PASTRIES

Reduce	Alternatives
Shortcrust	Filo
Puff	Wraps (Wholemeal & Maize Flour)
	Corn Dough

SUGAR

Sugar	Alternatives
White Refined Sugar	Brown Sugar
	Stevia
	Honey
	Maple Syrup
	Coconut Sugar

As I have mentioned many times, please try hard to reduce the amount of sugar in your diet.

SAUCES

Reduce	Alternatives
Creamy Hot Sauces (If possible)	Tabasco

Ketchup, Brown, Salad Cream, and Similar Condiments	Light Chilli Sauces & Flakes
Mayonnaise	Reduced Sugar/Fat Ketchups etc
	Reduced Fat Mayonnaise
	Vinaigrette
	Lemon & Olive Oil

Hot pepper sauce, we so dearly love, can contain excessive amounts of sodium (salt) so reduce the amount you use or try making your own healthier alternative.

SALT (SODIUM)

Reduce	Alternatives
All Purpose Seasoning	Paprika
Maggi Cubes	Curcumin (Turmeric)
Ready Packed Jerk Seasoning	Cayenne Pepper
Ready Packed Fish Seasoning	Cumin
Ready Packed Curry Powder	
Gravy Granules/Cubes	

I am, by no means, suggesting that you do not use the above items. Instead, make a conscious decision to reduce them, especially if you know that your meals have that salty rich flavour already.

Blending your own spices is also a great way to reduce the salt; however, I understand it can be time consuming or it's just something you don't and will not do. Using readymade shop bought seasoning is attractive and easy, just be mindful of how much you use and increase the flavour by adding some of the suggested alternatives that have lower sodium levels.

DESSERTS & SWEETS

Slowly Reduce	Alternatives
Cakes	Fruit
Sweet Pastries	Low Fat Yoghurts with Probiotics
Puddings	Low Fat Mousse
Ice Cream	Low Calorie Ice Cream
Sweets	
Chocolate	

DRINKS

Reduce	Alternatives
Alcohol	Water
Fizzy Drinks	Sugar Free Fizzy Drinks
Sugary Beverages	Low Calorie Tonic & Soda Water

Healthy Black Life

Fruit Juices

Caffeinated Drinks

Reduced Sugar Diluted Juices

Cranberry Juice

Herbal Teas

Drink more water!

I can't emphasise this enough, water is our miracle healer and it's generally free. Water flushes out the toxins in our body, maintains and balances our body fluids.

Always check the colour of your pee when you go to the toilet, as the colour will determine if and how much you are dehydrated. The rule of thumb is, the darker it is, the more dehydrated you are. That is why it is usually darker when we get up in the morning, because we haven't been drinking much fluid, if any, throughout the night. So if you like to start your day with a tea or coffee then try to add a tall glass of water. It will help to wake up your body and get you ready to start the day.

So if you like to start your day with a tea or coffee then try to add a tall glass of water...

Vegetables

One food group that seems to be missing from our diet (or is an afterthought) is good, wholesome regular vegetables. I'm not talking about yam, potato, or cassava but the more colourful vegetables that contain many macronutrients our body needs to stay energised and functional.

How much multi-coloured plant food is on your plate at mealtime?

Cultural Food Guide to Better Health

Fill one third of your plate with vegetables, or make sure this food group is larger than the rice...

Fill one third of your plate with vegetables, or make sure this food group is larger than the rice or potato starch-based portion of food on your plate. I believe this will increase your energy levels, give you that 'get up and go' feeling more often and help with weight management. Even frozen vegetables are great to eat, as they can cut down the preparation time and can be as nutritious as fresh vegetables.

I encourage you to make changes to your plate if you know that you do not eat enough vegetables. Salad is a great healthy accompaniment to your meal, such as cucumber, lettuce, tomatoes, etc. and contain mostly water.

Fibre (Complex Carbohydrates)

Fibre is important for your digestive system and helps keep you regular (if you know what I mean), this is because your body cannot digest it, so passes it out as waste. Fibre in our diet is necessary for regulating sugar levels as well as helping us stay more satisfied for longer after eating.

Healthy Black Life

Here are some of the best foods that are high in fibre

- Fruit and Vegetables
- Nuts
- Lentils
- Wholegrains
- Beans
- Popcorn
- Dried Fruit

Back in the 80's, high fibre diets were all the rage and everyone wanted to try this method of losing weight, even me. Yes, I was able to lose weight especially around my hips and thighs, however, too much fibre meant that my colon was working overtime because of the amount of waste I was producing and if I didn't drink enough water, I would become constipated. This led to many a tummy ache and even having a bout of colitis, so I would not recommend eating a diet high in fibre. However, it is important to include it in your diet.

Oily Fish

Fish is a good food source, so include fish weekly in your diet. However, be sure to include oily fish as it is great for supporting brain function and improving mood. Oily fish contains a rich source of Omega 3's helping to reduce the risk of Alzheimer's and Dementia as we age.

- Sardines
- Mackerel
- Salmon
- Herring
- Sprats

Oily fish contains a rich source of Omega 3's helping to reduce the risk of Alzheimer's and Dementia as we age.

I grew up on tinned sardines and continue to love them today. I tend to eat them as a snack, maybe with some salad and a cracker or even on its own. Sardines remain a staple food in black culture so keep on eating them and ensure you drain off the excess oil. There are many other varieties of tinned sardines available these days, including tomato, brine, pepper and so on, so be sure to make them a regular item in your kitchen.

Herbs & Spices

There are many powerful health benefits that are attached to herbs and spices. Here are a few to note and their benefits:

Turmeric	– anti-inflammatory
Curcumin	– contained in turmeric and is an antioxidant
Sage	– improves brain and memory function
Cayenne Pepper	– helps suppress appetite
Garlic	– helps maintain heart health

Healthy Black Life

Herbs and spices do much more than just enrich the flavours in our food, so continue to use them.

Fruit

The best way to eat fruit is in its natural form, rather than as a juice, as it's the best way for your body to maximise the vitamins and minerals they contain.

Diabetic Meal Guide

If you are or think you may be diabetic, be mindful of what is on your meal plate. Here are some tips to help balance your sugar levels.

Include

Vegetables & Salad
Include a good amount and a variety of colours to get the macronutrients your body needs to function well.

Drink Water
This is particularly important in the winter months as we tend to drink less.

Beans

Kidney, gungo, black eye, and others are a good source of fibre and protein.

Herbs

Fresh and dried herbs can have powerful health benefits.

Fruit

Be sure not to eat more than two servings a day because of the natural sugar they contain, as the glucose can spike insulin levels.

Here are some recommended fruits if you are diabetic:

- Blueberries
- Cherries
- Strawberries
- Apples
- Grapes
- Oranges
- Grapefruit
- Pear
- Peaches
- Kiwi

Healthy Black Life

Essential Vitamins and Minerals for Good Health

During the Covid-19 pandemic, the importance of **Vitamin D** was highlighted because of its ability to stimulate and strengthen our immune system. We absorb vitamin D through our skin by natural sunlight, and because of the beautiful, rich, dark colour we possess, our skin helps protect us from dangerous UV rays. Research suggests most people are deficient in vitamin D, especially in the winter as we spend more time

...black people are more at risk of vitamin D deficiency, as it takes longer for us to absorb the vitamin D from the sun because of the high levels of melanin in our skin.

inside and our daylight hours are shorter (in the UK). However, black people are more at risk of vitamin D deficiency, as it takes longer for us to absorb the vitamin D from the sun because of the high levels of melanin in our skin. This means it may be helpful to take this vitamin supplement in the winter months to boost our immune system, especially against viruses that thrive in the colder months. So going outside in the winter, even for a fifteen-minute walk, will help strengthen your immune system to fight off virus and infections. We can receive our dose of vitamin D even when there is cloud cover, so make an effort to keep yourself well and try not to hibernate in the winter.

The table below contains essential nutrients and their effect on the body. If you are not getting enough nutrients through your diet then an option is to take supplements.

However, the best way to get your vitamins and minerals is through your food, so try to incorporate the foods below into your diet.[1]

Vitamin	Benefits	Food Source
A	Immune system Vision Growth and development	Dairy & eggs Carrots Green leafy vegetables Sweet potatoes
B	Energy Brain function Vision Digestion Immune system Cell health	Seafood Poultry & meat Chickpeas Dairy & eggs Cereals with added vitamins Potatoes
C	Protects cells Immune system Tissue & wound healing	Fruit Vegetables
D (Important for Immunity)	Immune system Blood pressure regulator Nervous system Hormone production	Sunshine Fish & fish oils Eggs Added to dairy/cereals Mushrooms
E	Cell protection Immune system Blood vessel formation	Green vegetables Nuts & seeds Cereals & juice (vitamin E added)
K	Strengthen bones Blood clotting to stop excessive bleeding	Green vegetables

---

1 www.fda.gov/nutritioneducation

Healthy Black Life

Mineral	Benefits	Found in
Calcium	Blood clotting to stop excessive bleeding Blood vessel contract & restrict Nervous system Muscle use	Dairy Canned fish Green vegetables Added to cereals & orange & plant-based juices (soy, rice, almond)
Chloride	Digestion Balance acid Fluid balance Nervous system	Olives Rye Salt Vegetables (celery, tomatoes, lettuce)
Chromium	Insulin function Metabolism	Broccoli Fruit Juice Meat Spices Wholegrains
Copper	Cell health Energy Bone & tissue formation Iron Metabolism	Nuts & seeds Lentils Cocoa & chocolate Wholegrains Organ meat (liver)
Iodine	Production of red cells Wound healing Growth and development Reproduction Immune system	Dairy Fish Bread & cereals Potatoes Salt Turkey

Iron	Immune system	Green vegetables
	Energy	Meat & poultry & organ meat
	Growth & development	Fruit
	Reproduction	Beans
	Healing of wounds	Fish
		Eggs
		Wholegrains
		Soy products (tofu)
Magnesium	Blood sugar & pressure regulation	Avocado
	Hormone secretion	Fruit
	Heart rhythm	Green leafy vegetables
	Immune system	Diary
	Bone formation	Nuts
	Nervous system	Potatoes
		Wholegrains
Manganese	Metabolism	Nuts
	Wound healing	Beans
	Cartlidge & bone formation	Spinach
		Pineapple
		Sweet potatoes
Phosphorous	Energy	Dairy
	Bone formation	Meat & poultry
	Acid balance	Fish
		Nuts & seeds
Potassium	Blood pressure regulation	Fruit
	Carbohydrate metabolism	Beans
	Fluid balance	Dairy
	Heart	Fish
	Nervous system	Juices
	Muscle contraction	Vegetables

Healthy Black Life

Insulin-Like Growth Factor (IGF)

Let me ask you a question: Do you want to stay younger for longer? Do I hear a resounding 'yes'? This youth hormone (IGF) does just that; however, it's production naturally decreases in our bodies as we age. It is produced in our liver and studies have shown it improves cognitive function and blood flow to the brain. Thankfully, there are certain foods and vitamins that help to optimise this youth hormone which, in a nutshell,

...there are certain foods and vitamins that help to optimise this youth hormone which, in a nutshell, delays the symptoms of aging.

delays the symptoms of aging. If you would like to stay youthful for as long as possible, take a look at the vitamins and minerals below and the different foods[2] which will help optimize the production of IGF:

- **Zinc**

    Spinach

    Mushrooms

    Cashew Nuts

    Oysters

    Pumpkin Seeds

    Grass Fed Beef

---

2 https://www.optimallivingdynamics.com/blog/increase-insulin-like-growth-factor-igf-1-levels

- **Protein**
  - Meat
  - Dairy
  - Eggs
  - Broccoli
  - Nuts & Seeds
  - Soya
  - Beans & Pulses
- **Blueberries**
- **Vitamin C**
  - Fruit
  - Vegetables
- **Magnesium**
  - Spinach
  - Chard
  - Pumpkin Seeds
  - Almonds
  - Avocado
  - Dark Chocolate
  - Bananas
- **Selenium**
  - Brazil Nuts
  - Wild Seafood
  - Grass Fed Meat
  - Pastured Chicken and Eggs

Healthy Black Life

- **Cinnamon**
- **Vitamin D**
    Sunshine

    Eggs

    Red Meat
- **Dried plums**

Summary

I have laid out lots of information in this chapter to help you start on your healthier black life journey through what we eat and how much.

Advice includes:

- Eating Tips
- Healthier Cooking Options
- Healthier Alternative Dietary Options
- Additional Food to Add to Your Diet
- Diabetic Food Guidance
- Essential Vitamins and Minerals
- Hormone Impact

I hope this information encourages you to consider the following steps you can make to a healthier, happier you. Choose where you would like to start and make that one change and when you feel ready, try adding another. Your journey takes time, so give yourself the mental and emotional space to adjust.

Your journey takes time, so give yourself the mental and emotional space to adjust.

Chapter Six

———◆◆◆———

You Matter (Body & Mind)

Through the Years (Age)

How many have heard the phrase, 'age is but a number'? This is a good positive phrase to live by, however, we do age, and biologically, our body eventually becomes less efficient and starts to wear out. So, age is *not* just a number! Let's review the biological stages of aging and its effect on us.

Young Adults (18-30)

In young adulthood, you are generally in your prime. Your body is now fully developed, your energy levels are high, and you are ready to take on the world. Nothing can stop you going after your dreams. Your mindset shouts that you are free to step into new, exciting opportunities without the stumbling block of fear. It's natural to think that young people are more active than any other adult age group, however, the advancements in technology over the last two decades have seen young people engrossed in electronic devices. Many are sitting and staring at an oblong shaped device, enjoying the delights of checking out what everyone and anyone in the world is posting on social media, playing games, or watching boxsets for hours on end. I must admit, I am concerned about the impact technology is having on the physical and mental well-being of this generation.

Adults (31 – 45)

As we cruise through these years, lifestyle has a bigger impact on how the body is dealing with life. We generally have an established way of living through work, family, social networks and, more importantly, our nutrition and fitness regimes. In this age group, we are more likely to become set in our ways—just doing life. But it can also be the age where we may pause and take stock of life and decide it's time to make some changes. Our habitual thinking, however, can make it harder to motivate oneself to make the relevant changes necessary, especially if we believe the journey to better health will be long and not much fun. We may also be suffering from physical ailments or health issues which could be impacting our quality of life.

Older Adults (46 – 60)

Okay, this is my age group, so I can speak from life right now. Generally, this is the age when our hormones have a major impact on our body as we move out of the procreation age and start to recognise our body is slowing down. Women feel the full force of these changes with the onset of Peri-menopause and Menopause, and men experience a drop in testosterone levels. Our body shape changes, as our waistline starts to thicken, and we find many more grey hairs. You may also notice that your energy levels reduce, and therefore, adopt a more sedentary lifestyle. As we age, our 'youth hormone' IGF-1 (as mentioned in the previous chapter) begins to reduce more rapidly, which speeds up the aging process.

Seniors (65+)

When we reach this age group, we generally have reached the end of our working career and are ready to slow down. You may be enjoying family life with adult children and watching the grandchildren grow. The body may start to feel tired easier, and aches and pains around the joints

What you experience as you age is determined by the physical and mental choices you make—no matter how old you are.

may have set in, especially in the wintertime. You may be experiencing more disease or sickness and taking medication on a regular basis; or indeed you may be as healthy as you were in your forties depending on your life choices thus far. At this stage of life, you may be motivated to start looking at making changes that will improve your health and slow down the aging process. Or you may be content to just be able to get out of bed in the morning. This is perfectly normal, as you probably feel like you have done your share of working and taking care of family, and you just want to relax and enjoy life. Those in this age bracket may travel and take more holidays, health permitting, now that the children are grown and have families of their own.

What you experience as you age is determined by the physical and mental choices you make—no matter how old you are.

The Shape of You

What words come to mind when you think of the body shape of black men and women? The words that come to my mind are SHAPELY, CURVY, STRONG, and MUSCULAR.

When I was growing up in the town of Dagenham in the UK, I noticed that my shape was different to my fellow white skinned friends at school. My hips seemed to be growing at a greater rate than the rest of me, and I thought my 'booty' could be seen from the moon! Nowadays, young people are paying thousands of pounds or spending the most amount of time in the gym trying to achieve this look. But back then, I was frustrated because clothes wouldn't fit my lower half well, especially denim jeans. Clothes were made for the mass market of the british figure, which lacked shape and curvature. So, not only did I stand out in school because of the colour of my skin in the 1980s, but I also had a different shape. Lord, have mercy!

Our bodies are all different shapes and sizes. For this reason, it's helpful to know more about our own particular shape to establish what works for each of us when looking to make improvements to our health and fitness levels. This will also help you to understand what is achievable in terms of how you would like to look.

Let's take a glance at different frames and body types and how they can impact our health.

Body Frame

Male

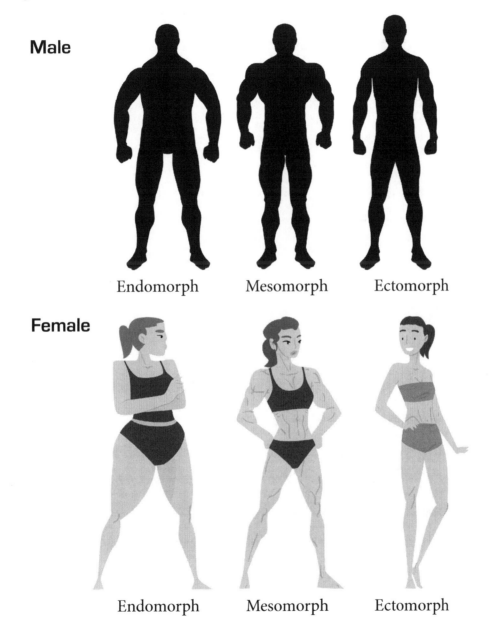

Endomorph   Mesomorph   Ectomorph

Female

Endomorph   Mesomorph   Ectomorph

You Matter (Body & Mind)

Endomorph

This body shape is what I would call full. An endomorph can be short or tall and have a thick waist and a block type body. Sometimes you can feel that you put on weight by just glancing at food, let alone eating it. You can have good muscle mass, but this can also be accompanied by a degree of fat which you may find hard to shift.

Mesomorph

The structure of a mesomorph is what I would call shapely; shoulders are wide, and your waist is smaller. You're basically the average body shape that can wear muscle and fat pretty equally. When you are ready to start an exercise regime, you can probably see results quickly, however, don't be fooled—you can also pack on the pounds if you have a very good relationship with bad food.

Ectomorph

This is the smaller of body frames which is generally slim and has little shape. You can be short or tall, but your levers (limbs) are long. You can find it challenging to put on weight or increase muscle mass, regardless of what you eat and physical exercise.

Did you identify with a particular frame? You may even find similarities with more than one body frame, but you will generally know which one is more dominant for you.

Body Type

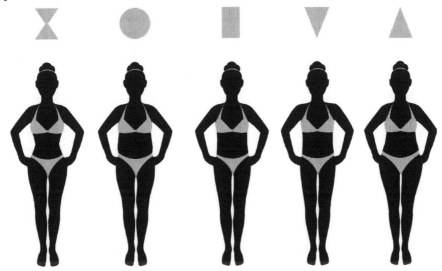

Female Body Types

Us ladies have a number of body types we can identify with, as you can see from the diagram. The different shapes[1] are largely due to the fat distribution in our bodies, however, keep in mind you may be a mixture of two or three different types. As you read on, consider what category/categories your body is generally geared towards.

Hourglass – Fat is developed on the chest area, with a thinner waist and then fat distribution around the hips. This shape is known to be the healthiest of all the body shapes and does not associate with many health risks. However, fat can still develop around vital organs (visceral fat) as well as stomach fat.

---

1 https://www.livestrong.com/article/13720203-body-shape-composition-health/

Apple – Body fat gathers around the upper body, especially the waistline. The apple shape has more of a tendency to produce this visceral fat which surrounds the organs, which means this shape is at a higher risk of developing disease.

Straight – There is more of an even distribution of fat around the body, and though the fat is not as visible in a particular area, it does not mean that fat around the organs doesn't exist. Because of the lack of body mass, people with this shape are at risk of developing osteoporosis due to a lack of bone density.

The Inverted Triangle – The main distinction with this body type is that the shoulders will be wider than the hips, but this body type shares characteristics with the others. Models and athletes generally have this shape, with the addition of long legs and a defined waistline. If body fat forms, it will generally sit on the upper body, which, again, can increase the risk of visceral fat.

Pear – I would associate my body type as this one, with body fat sitting on the hips and thighs. As the fat targets the lower body, there is less risk in developing disease because the vital organs are in the upper body. However, pear shape people may suffer more joint issues because of the extra lower body weight.

Did you identify your body type?

Healthy Black Life

Looking at your body composition can help you understand potential health risks and where you may need to focus your attention when it comes to adjusting your lifestyle and diet.

Remember this:

We do not all look the same and nor should we. This book is about improving your health, not about making you lose a stone in 6 weeks. Let's keep it real and understand that some of us will not look like a size 4 model after losing weight nor may we want to. The variety of shapes and sizes we come in add variety to life, so we must find acceptance and contentment in whichever body frame and shape we fit, and from this platform, live our healthiest and best life. We can all make improvements to our health by taking one simple step at a time.

Looking at your body composition can help you understand potential health risks...

Your fitness expectations and goals should fit within realistic outcomes, therefore improvement for you, however small, is what matters.

Body Weight

The term obese is used by medical professionals to indicate body weight is too high in comparison to an individual's height, and this is determined by calculating our Body

Mass Index (BMI). However, there is a problem with this method, as body weight does not differentiate between fat and muscle. So, a burly 6 foot, muscular, 17 stone rugby player or a thick built, black bodybuilder who is as strong as an ox can have a similar BMI as a sedentary, overweight person who has a much higher percentage of body fat.

Have you ever heard the phrase, 'Muscle weighs more than fat'? What it means is, muscle is much denser than fat, so when you touch muscle, it is generally harder, and fat is much softer. If you put 1kg of muscle on a weighing scale and then weigh out 1kg of fat, the mass of fat will be that much larger than the muscle mass even though they weigh the same. If you have good, developed muscles, then your BMI will probably be on the high side. However, this would not be a clear indicator of being overweight. In contrast, most people do not have a firm, hard, muscular built body, so this method is a general indicator of a healthy or unhealthy weight for the average individual.

...we have greater bone density than white people...

It is also important to note that we have greater bone density than white people, which now makes perfect sense due to the lack of black international swimmers across the planet as well as a lack of interest in taking to the water in general. I have heard friends say they feel like a brick or a piece of lead when they swim and struggle to keep their bodies afloat. This is especially true for those who have well developed muscles. Have you ever felt like this? I have; swimming for me always seems more of a struggle, hence I find other ways to exercise, even though I quite like being in water.

Healthy Black Life

Just over a year ago I visited my new dentist to refit my crown, which had fallen out, however, instead of putting it back in, suggested I have the remnants of the tooth removed. I reluctantly agreed to have the extraction, thinking it was the right thing to do for my dental health.

On the day of the removal, as fit and strong as my dentist looked, and after numerous numbing injections, he could not get the remainder of my tooth out. At one point, I thought he was going to climb on to the dentist chair and anchor his feet on the sides as he was drilling and yanking me about. He ended up taking out little slivers of it as my tooth shattered into pieces in my gum. When he finally gave up and asked me to rinse out my mouth, he said that my jawbone was very strong, and that black people in general have dense bones. He would have to send me to hospital to have the remainder of the tooth removed. My recovery from that experience I found unbearable, and the gum took weeks to heal. Hence, I haven't been back and it's been fine ever since.

Weight Management

Our total body weight consists of our bones, muscles, organs, ligaments, tendons, skin, and fat, as well as water, which surprisingly, makes up around 60% of our weight. If you have ever been on a weight loss programme, you may have witnessed a dramatic reduction in weight over a relatively short space of time, which is very encouraging when you are trying to change habits and improve your health. The main reason for this

Keep a food and exercise diary as writing down your progress helps to stay accountable.

is that the change to your diet can cause the body to drain extra water from your cells first. Weight loss may then start to slow as the body starts to break down fat.

HBL Steps

- Have a goal weight you would like to achieve but keep it realistic
- Give yourself time to reach your goal
- Set fortnightly or monthly goals to help you stay on track
- Keep a food and exercise diary as writing down your progress helps to stay accountable
- Look for an item of clothing you have, but is too tight to wear. Hang it somewhere you can see it daily to remind you of your goals and try it on periodically to help measure your progress
- To help keep you motivated, ask a family member or friend to lose weight with you so you can cheer each other on for every successful step, however small
- Support and encourage each other, especially on bad days
- Make time to prepare meals

There are many reasons why your body weight can plateau or fluctuate when choosing to lose weight, so don't be too discouraged if the scales are being unkind, especially when

Healthy Black Life

you believe you have been doing everything right. Focus on how you look in the mirror and how you feel and fit in your clothes rather than what the scales say.

If you exercise, your body shape might be positively changing more than your body weight. For example, if your workouts focus on building muscle mass and you regularly lift heavy weights (especially all you man dem!), then you may experience a better body shape but not much movement in your weight. In fact, your weight could even increase.

Where's Your Head At? (Mindset)

...how you think will surely have a direct impact on your health and fitness.

Space…the Final Frontier! I am referring to the space between your ears, which is where your precious brain is located. A complex piece of your anatomy which is the nerve centre of your whole being, and it is this head mass that will determine how you live your life. Your genetics, family, culture, environment, experiences and what you feed on mentally, will effectively contribute to your thought process.

Your mind is connected to everything you do, even when you act spontaneously, for instance, moving a limb or shifting your eyes. Whether you are conscious of it or not, whatever you do comes from your brain. That is how amazing and complex your brain matter is, and with a little understanding of how you process thought and action, it will help direct your life in a positive way. Your brain takes in new information throughout life and some learn quicker than others…and that's fine. But how you think will surely have a direct impact on your health and fitness.

You Matter (Body & Mind)

What you watch, listen to, eat, and do will also impact how you feel. More than ever, people are struggling with mental health issues as the impact of the Covid-19 pandemic unfolds. People have increasingly spent time in isolation, shut in with their TV and social media devices that have been feeding them far too much fear and negativity.

Do I value my mental health?

If you said yes to this question, what choices are you making in life that suggests this is the case?

If no, then what are you doing that demonstrates you do not value your mental health?

Here are some activities to consider to balance or improve your mental health:

HBL Steps

- Go for a walk where you are surrounded by nature, like a local park, green space, or countryside
- Think about what you are grateful for when you wake in the morning and count your blessings
- Choose your conversations wisely and speak positively instead of negatively
- Watch lighthearted TV that makes you laugh

Healthy Black Life

- Do not spend too much time watching or listening to the news or chat shows about current affairs
- Listen to music you enjoy
- Read a lighthearted book
- Exercise and meditate
- Have a nice soak in a bubble bath once in a while
- Book yourself a massage or purchase massage equipment/devices
- Go for a swim at your local pool or in the sea if you live near the coast when the weather is warm
- Make time to relax
- Pamper yourself
- Focus on positive thoughts and steer away from negative thoughts
- Have fun playing games with family and friends
- Spend quality time with those you love
- Try to maintain a good work/life balance

Now ask yourself the following questions to help pinpoint the areas of your life you want or need to address:

1. Are you happy with your current health right now?
2. Do you think positively about yourself most of the time?
3. Do you wake up looking forward to the day?

4. Do you feel good most of the time?

5. Do you smile or laugh a lot?

6. Do you make time to do some form of exercise?

7. Do you find yourself sitting for most of the day?

8. Are you tired most of the time?

9. Do you sleep well?

Pause and think about your answers, then make the necessary changes one step at a time.

Chapter Seven

❖◆◆❖

The Importance of Movement (Exercise)

One thing the Covid-19 pandemic highlighted is the importance of healthy lungs. Exercising our cardiovascular system will strengthen our heart and lungs by increasing the airflow through breathing deeper. Your heart is a muscle, therefore, it needs exercise to help pump blood to every part of your body, from the top of your head right down to your baby toes. The stronger your heart, the more protection you have when your body is under viral attack.

The stronger your heart, the more protection you have when your body is under viral attack.

So, it is important to:

- Breathe deeply to oxygenate our blood and increase lung capacity
- Exercise the heart muscle to transport the blood, which feeds our body and carries out day-to-day maintenance

Do you know the phrase 'Whatever you put in, you get out'? This statement is about quantity, or measure, and in the health and fitness world, relates to the effort necessary to see positive change to better health, and it does take effort. So, try to get your head in the game, because a positive mental attitude will sustain you on the bad days.

Hear this! Exercise does not only have to take place in the gym.

Movement is key to looking after your body, and how much you move matters greatly. The important thing is that you try to move the whole body regularly. And if this helps at all, you don't have to call this exercise (if the word makes you feel nauseous!).

The largest muscle in our body is our quadricep (thigh), so leg movement is a good way to work the heart and strengthen the lungs (through deeper breathing). The larger the muscle you move, the stronger the heart needs to pump blood and oxygen to that area. The speed of the movement will impact our heart rate (beat) and our metabolism, which will help burn calories and assist in weight management.

Hear this! Exercise does not only have to take place in the gym.

Movement at Home

Question…What are you doing at home?

If you find it hard to motivate yourself to exercise, just increase your movement at home instead.

Which of these statements would you say relates to your lifestyle?

> I spend a lot of time sitting in front of the telly.
>
> I can't sit for long, so I'm always getting up finding things to do.

There are many ways to add more movement to your home life. Here are some suggestions:

Play Up-Tempo Music

Music and dancing are embedded in black culture and is an important part of our lives, as it accompanies social events, celebrations, and brings enjoyment. From the drums rooted deep in the African continent and the vibrance of afro beats, to the majestic soca and calypso music that manifests from the shores of the Caribbean. The energy our music creates has influenced countries all over the world. Dance brings people together in a dynamic atmosphere, creating interaction and a whole lot of smiling and movement. As a Zumba instructor, so many people have shared with me how much they enjoy taking part in my classes as it's a fun way to exercise. So, dancing is a great way to add movement to your day, burn some calories, and raise your heart rate. Many a night I put my headphones in my ears, lower the lights, and silently dance my socks off around the living room, often late into the night. Don't just leave dancing to social occasions—put on some of your favourite tunes, dance around your home, and 'get down' on a regular basis. It will also help lift your mood and contribute to good health.

> **Don't just leave dancing to social occasions—put on some of your favourite tunes, dance around your home...**

Regularly Walk or Jog Upstairs

If you have stairs in your home, make a conscious effort to walk up and down them regularly to add more movement and train your heart muscle. Do what you can; start with what feels comfortable, then add more movement, for example, lifting your knees higher and swinging your arms. You can even increase the speed at which you climb, which will increase your breathing and heart rate. If you don't have stairs but have a doorstep, use this to do step ups instead.

Increase Housework

Cleaning adds movement to your day, so if you are not sold on the whole exercise thing, increasing home chores on a weekly basis is another way to burn a few extra calories.

Healthy Black Life

Here are some home cleaning chores you can do regularly to increase movement:

- Hoovering/Sweeping
- Mopping the Floor
- Dusting
- Deep Cleaning
- Window Cleaning
- Washing Up
- Emptying Dishwasher
- Cleaning Out Wardrobes
- Tidying Garden Shed
- Gardening

...increasing home chores on a weekly basis is another way to burn a few extra calories.

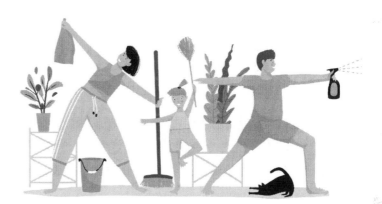

If you are only using your upper body as you clean, march your feet on the spot or kick your heels up towards your bottom to add movement.

Think of extra ways you can move your body to increase and exaggerate the movements. Putting on some of your favourite high tempo music as mentioned before, will inspire you to move more while you push the hoover or broom around the living room or polish the shelves.

The Importance of Movement (Exercise)

I'm sure there are many more activities you can think of doing in your home, but make sure you open the windows to let in fresh air (especially if there is dust in the air or if you are using chemicals to clean) and wear a mask if you have breathing difficulties, allergies, or asthma.

HBL Steps

- Listen to your favourite music and dance around your home more often for improved mental and physical health
- Walk upstairs at home on purpose or do step-ups on a step to increase your heart rate
- Increase movement whilst doing housework
- Put on music when cleaning to encourage you to move more.

Note: To stay accountable, if possible, purchase a device to wear on your wrist (for example a Fitbit) to monitor how many steps you are achieving per day. You can add target steps to your device to ensure you are increasing movement and stay on track.

Movement At Work

How much you move at work is determined by how physical your job is, for instance, working in a busy kitchen versus working an office job. See the suggestions below on how to increase or decrease your movement during the day based on various career sectors.

Office/Home Working

If you work at a desk most of the day, try to get on your feet and go for a walk around the office/home to wake up your body, even if it is just for 5 minutes. It's good to get the flow of blood moving around with some movement with 5-10 minutes of stretching your limbs. While you are sitting at your desk, you can lift your feet in a stepping motion under the desk to work your lower body. You can make up whatever movement you like as long it does not feel too uncomfortable. You may even want to move your chair out of the way to stand up and work if you can for a certain amount of time. The important thing is to try to consciously move more often.

If possible, get up and walk around every 30 minutes, even if it's just for a few minutes.

HBL Steps

- If possible, get up and walk around every 30 minutes, even if it's just for a few minutes
- Stretch for 5-10 minutes
- Lift your feet up and down in a marching motion while sitting at your desk
- Stand up and work for a while

Retail and Hospitality Industry

You may spend a lot of your day on your feet, working in retail or hospitality, which is great for movement, as long as you are not standing in one spot for long periods of time. If you are sitting on a checkout/reception/customer service desk etc, you can keep your lower body moving by lifting your feet in a stepping motion and rolling your ankles now and then. If you are standing for a considerable amount of time, try to alleviate pressure on your legs by making sure you sit down during your break.

HBL Steps

- If standing still for long periods of time, move your legs every so often, i.e. marching on the spot
- If sitting at a desk, lift your feet alternately and roll ankles once in a while
- Sit down when you can to relieve the pressure on your legs and joints

A high percentage of the black and Asian community work in the Care sector...

Care Workers

A high percentage of the black and Asian community work in the Care sector, especially our National Health Service (NHS) in the UK. This can be a very physical, stressful job and can draw long working hours and as a result, can impact mental health and energy levels. Therefore, finding time to relax the body and mind is very important to maintain good health.

Healthy Black Life

You can do this by listening to relaxing music, watching easy TV, reading, and even adding meditation and exercise such as yoga to your week.

HBL Steps

- To reduce physical stress levels, sit/lay down to relax the body
- To reduce mental stress levels, listen to relaxing music, try yoga with meditation, watch easy TV, or read

Driver

If your job involves sitting in a vehicle most of the day, it's very difficult to suggest extra movement; however, when you are on a break, be conscious about moving your body. If it is safe to do so, get out of the vehicle and have a walk around or go for a stroll and add some simple stretches. After work, engage in a hobby that requires a lot of movement, or exercise, before you sit down again for the evening.

HBL Steps

- On breaks, go for a walk, or stretch, even if it's just for 10 minutes
- After work, engage in a hobby that requires a lot of movement
- Exercise

Chapter Eight

———— ✦ ————

Let's Get Physical

Walking

Going outside is a great way to add more movement into your day and to get fresh air into your lungs, so try to make time to go for a walk. It can be in a local park or just around your neighbourhood, and if all you can manage is a gentle walk, that's absolutely fine. Increasing your pace to a power walk occasionally during your walk is a good way to raise your heart rate. This will cause you to breathe heavier and allow more blood and oxygen to reach the muscles.

Benefits of Walking

- Helps weight management
- Strengthens muscles and joints
- Encourages you to breathe deeper
- Enlarges and strengthens lung capacity with increased walking pace

Increasing your pace to a power walk occasionally during your walk is a good way to raise your heart rate.

- Strengthens heart muscle and cardiovascular system (breath)
- Lifts your mood
- Increases Vitamin D strengthening your immune system
- Walking in green spaces helps to improve mental health

Try this basic HBL Walking Workout:

- Go for a walk for a minimum of 20 minutes, 3-4 times a week
- Speed up and slow down your walking pace to increase heart rate
- If you are able, turn your walk in to a power walk/jog from time to time
- Take a bottle of water with you
- Exaggerate arm motion to work upper body
- Take a rest when and if you feel you need it
- Ask a family member or friend to join you

...most adults do not breathe efficiently, therefore shallow breathing is much more common.

Breathing

Did you know that most adults do not breathe efficiently, therefore shallow breathing is much more common. Most of us don't really give breathing a second thought as it is a natural unconscious function our body just performs. However, the effectiveness of breathing not only strengthens the heart muscle and lungs but also increases blood circulation and oxygenates the blood.

One thing I continually remind my clients and members to do in class is to breathe. 'Take a big breath in through your nose and blow out through your mouth.' Breathing well helps our muscle and lung performance during exercise. Sometimes, I find my clients yawning as they exercise, which is an indication they need more oxygen. Thus, the body automatically triggers yawning as a means to take in more air.

MyFitnessPal[1] states these benefits to deep breathing:

- *Expands lung capacity*
- *Minimises pain (ex. breathing techniques during labour)*
- *Reduces stress and anxiety*
- *Improves energy and mood*
- *Brings peace of mind*

All of these are important in enhancing health and well-being, physically and mentally. Yoga engages the unity of the mind and body to reach a sense of calm and relaxation whilst breathing through the movements and positions.

---

1 https://blog.myfitnesspal.com

Headspace.com[2] states breathing effectively can also

- *Reduce stress levels and the hormone cortisol*
- *Lower blood pressure*
- *Reduce your heart rate*
- *Relax muscles*

Breathing well has many benefits and is something we rarely consider in our day...

Breathing well has many benefits and is something we rarely consider in our day to day unless we are considerably overweight, suffer with allergies such as hay fever and asthma, or have a cardiovascular disease, for example, Chronic Obstructive Pulmonary Disease (COPD).

Belly breathing is easy to do and very relaxing. Try this basic exercise anytime you need to relax or relieve stress.

Breathing Exercise[3]
- *Sit or lie flat in a comfortable position*
- *Put one hand on your belly just below your ribs and the other hand on your chest*
- *Take a deep breath in through your nose, and let your belly push your hand out*
  Your chest should not move

---

2 https://headspace.com

3 https://www.uofmhealth.org

Healthy Black Life

- *Breathe out through pursed lips as if you were whistling. Feel the hand on your belly go in, and use it to push all the air out*
- *Do this exercise 3 to 10 times. Take your time with each breath*
- *Notice how you feel at the end of the exercise*

I love the way focusing on my breathing makes me feel. It completely relaxes my body and mind, enabling me to feel centred and peaceful. Give it a try!

Home Exercise

This is not a sprint to better health, it's a steady transition to new and healthier habits.

There are many exercises you can try at home to strengthen your body, increase your fitness levels, and/or reduce your weight to improve health.

If you are new to exercise or have health concerns, please consult your health practitioner before engaging in any fitness programme.

I encourage you to make a plan, which will help you stick with a regular exercise routine. Do whatever you are able to do, taking small, simple steps but stay consistent. The important thing is that you do something, even if you start with just a 15 minute workout. Take your time and get used to some of the exercises before you add more. This is not a sprint to better health, it's a steady transition to new and healthier habits. To help prevent injury, ensure you warm up and cool down before and after you exercise.

HBL Steps

- Consult your GP if you have health issues or if new to exercise
- Make a plan to work out on certain days of the week for a set amount of time around 15-40 minutes
- Take your time and increase intensity gradually
- Stay consistent

Simple Yoga

Yoga is a great way to start exercising as it comes with many benefits that can be foundational to improved health.

Benefits of Yoga

- Increases flexibility
- Improves breathing
- Increases strength and balance
- Reduces arthritic joint pain
- Reduces back complaints
- Increases lung health
- Relaxes the mind
- Reduces stress

Next are some yoga poses to try at home, so start with the easier poses and in time, add poses you find more challenging.

As you flow through the movements, breathe in when your body is closed (i.e. limbs closer to body) and breathe out when your body opens out. Try to keep steady breaths in and out as you hold the poses.

Select 10-15 poses, perform 2 sets holding each pose for 20 seconds.

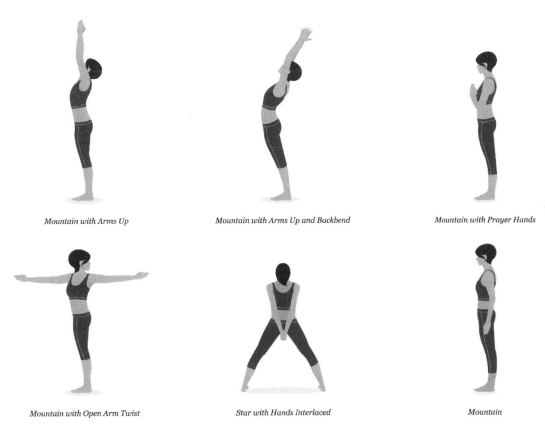

Mountain with Arms Up   *Mountain with Arms Up and Backbend*   *Mountain with Prayer Hands*

Mountain with Open Arm Twist   *Star with Hands Interlaced*   *Mountain*

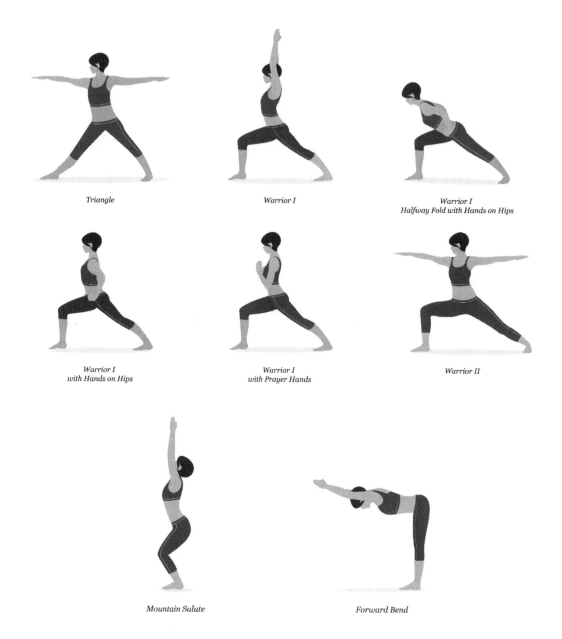

Triangle

Warrior I

Warrior I
Halfway Fold with Hands on Hips

Warrior I
with Hands on Hips

Warrior I
with Prayer Hands

Warrior II

Mountain Salute

Forward Bend

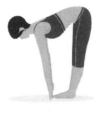

Halfway Lift

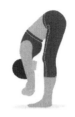

Rag Doll

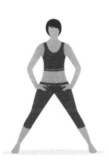

Star with Hands on Hips

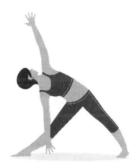

Triangle

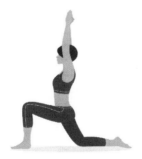

Crescent Lunge on the Knee

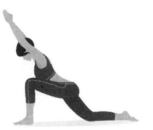

*Crescent Lunge Halfway Fold
on the Knee*

Let's Get Physical

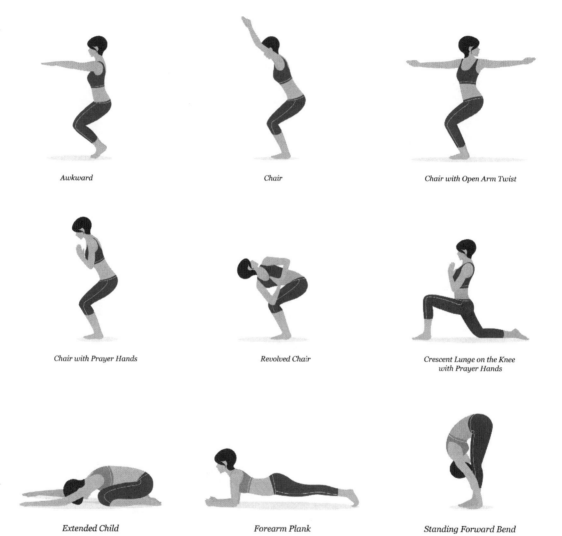

Awkward

Chair

Chair with Open Arm Twist

Chair with Prayer Hands

Revolved Chair

Crescent Lunge on the Knee
with Prayer Hands

Extended Child

Forearm Plank

Standing Forward Bend

Healthy Black Life

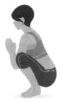

Garland

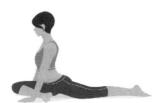

Half Pigeon

Happy Baby

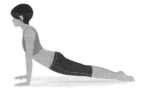

Upward-Facing Dog

Hero

Half Lotus Twist

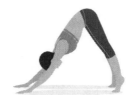

Downward-Facing Dog with Toe Raises

Let's Get Physical

Chair Yoga

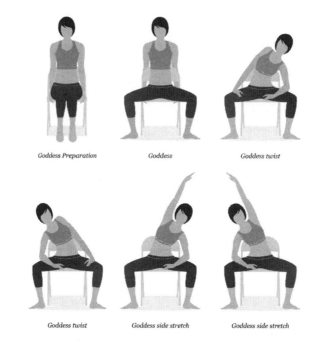

Goddess Preparation

Goddess

Goddess twist

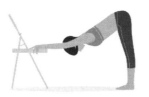

Goddess twist

Goddess side stretch

Goddess side stretch

Wide Downward Facing Dog

Supported Pyramid

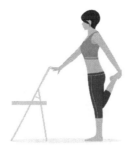

Thigh Stretch

Low Lunge

Healthy Black Life

Warm Up

Before you start any of the following workouts, it is important to warm up to prepare your body for more movement. By warming up your joints and muscles, you reduce the risk of injury as well as gradually increasing your heart rate without shocking the system by doing too much too soon.

A warm up lasts for around 5-10 minutes and movements can consist of a power walk and/or a combination of the warm up movements below:

- March on the spot using your arms in a running motion
- Arms by your side and then swing back and forth and add single arm circles
- Kick your heels up to your bottom
- Alternate tapping your heels (lift your knee up and tap inside of opposite foot)
- Gentle squats (do not go down too low)
- Bicep curls with alternating heel presses

Check out the Healthy Black Life YouTube channel where you will find demonstrations of these warm up and cool down stretches as well as much more to support you in your better health journey. Bear in mind the yoga poses on the previous pages can also be used as a cool down after any workout.

Check out the Healthy Black Life YouTube channel...

Let's move on to some more vigorous exercise. Just remember to do what you can, as something is better than nothing.

Home Workout

Choose 8-12 exercises

Duration: 20-30 seconds

Sets: 2-3

Rest: 3-5 minutes between sets

High Knees

This is a running motion which can be performed slowly or can be sped up to add a bounce.

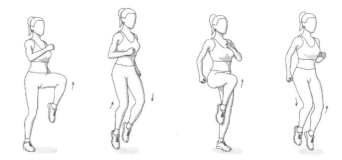

Side Lunges

As you step to the side, bend your knees, and push your bottom back and down. Keep your knees behind toes as you bend.

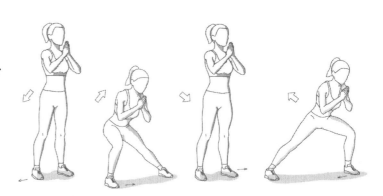

Healthy Black Life

Mountain Climbers

Alternate lifting your leg and opposite arm up as if you are climbing.

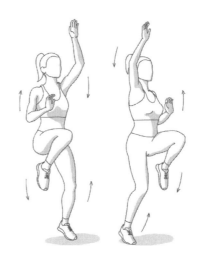

Push Ups

Options:

Beginners – keep knees on floor

Intermediate - full push up on toes, push your chest away from the floor

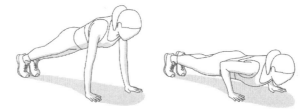

The following 3 exercises are for your Core (abs and back) and are best suited towards the end of your set as they can exhaust your waist area, affecting posture when performing other exercises.

Lying Leg Raises

Try to keep your heels off the floor when lowering legs, then slowly raise them again.

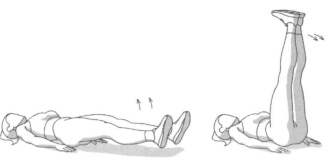

Seated Crunch

Try to keep your heels off the floor when legs are out but touch your heels down if you struggle with this one.

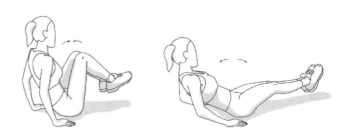

V Sit

Hold this position for between 10-40 seconds. The easier option is to place your feet on the floor and lean back.

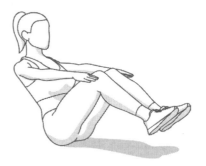

Healthy Black Life

Wide Squat Deadlift with Dumbbell

Feel your body weight through your heels as you squat. You do not have to hold a weight.

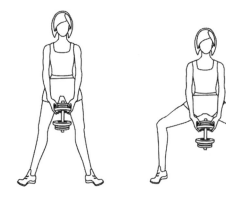

Squat Jumps

This is a more advanced move. Sit back in a squat position and focus on your body weight pushing through your heels. Keep your knees behind your toes then jump into the air. If you suffer with knee problems take out the jump and stick with normal squats.

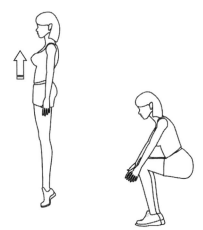

Single Leg Lift

Keep the knee of the standing leg slightly bent while you lift other leg back. Change and do this on the opposite leg after at least 4-8 lifts.

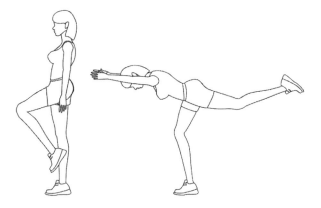

Step Ups

Step up and down. This exercise can be performed on a doorstep or on the bottom step of a staircase.

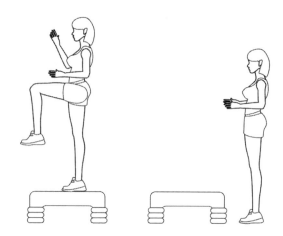

Tricep Dips

Fingers facing forward with bottom close to bench/step (or firm sofa) as you lower your body towards the floor until your arm is at a right angle at the elbow, then push up.

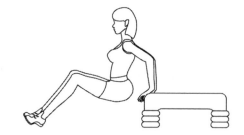

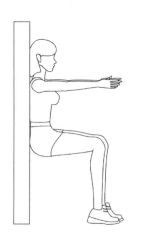

Wall Sit

Find a wall and sit with your back pushing into it with your tailbone tucked under. Hold this position for 20-40 seconds. If arms get tired, rest them on your thighs.

Healthy Black Life

Lunge Kicks

Starting in a lunge position, pick up the back leg and kick it through. For balance, you may want to hold on to the arm of a sofa.

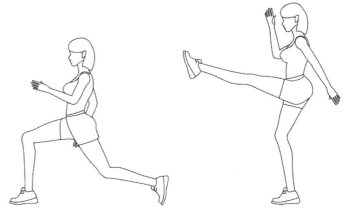

Floor Runs

Alternate lifting your knees up towards arms.

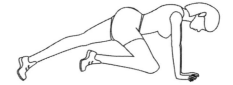

Lying Leg Lifts

You can do this exercise without the band, keeping your hips forward as you lift your leg.

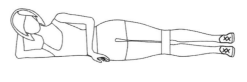

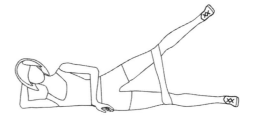

Let's Get Physical

Shoulder Bridge

Legs hip width apart and push pelvis up as you lift your bottom off the floor.

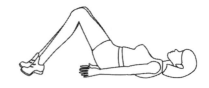

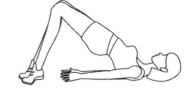

Reverse Lunge

Ensure you step the leg back and not forward when attempting a lunge to reduce risk of knee injury. Lower the knee towards the floor (but don't touch floor), then place feet back together and repeat on other side.

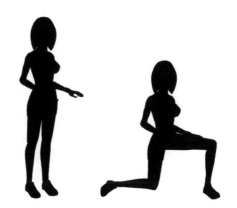

Side Arm Raises

You can do this exercise with or without holding a weight/bottle of water and keep your elbows slightly bent as you raise arms.

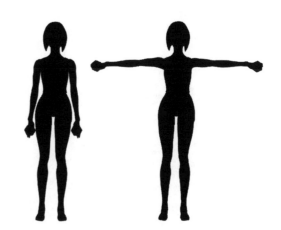

128

Side Leg Raises

Hold on to the back of a chair or a table and try to keep your body upright while swinging the leg out and up.

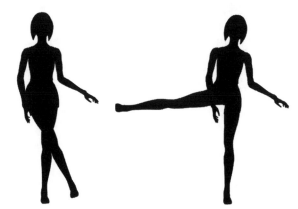

Lunge Jump

From a lunge position, swing knee through to the front and jump up, then replace the same leg behind again. Alternatively, you can remove the jump as this is an advanced exercise. Change leg after 20 seconds.

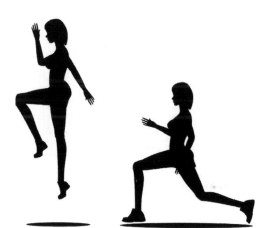

Swimmers

Alternate lifting arms and legs up and down at the same time whilst raising your chest off the floor.

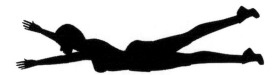

Overhead Shoulder Press

Use small weights or small bottles of water and push weights upwards. If you prefer, do this without a weight to begin with.

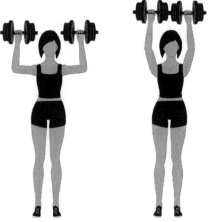

Side Bends

Stand with a slight bend in both knees and tuck your pubic bone under. Then, alternate side bends, keeping the lower body still when lowering arm down the leg. Using a weight is optional.

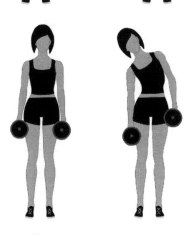

Squats

From a standing position with feet hip width apart push your bottom back and down, feeling the weight of your body through your heels and keep your knees behind your toes as you squat down.

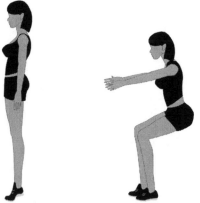

Healthy Black Life

Kneeling Kickbacks

Start in a tabletop position with knees directly under hips and shoulders over wrists. You can also try bringing your chest closer to the floor and rest on your forearms instead of your hands. Swing knee up and then down without touching the floor and repeat. Change side after 10-15 kickbacks.

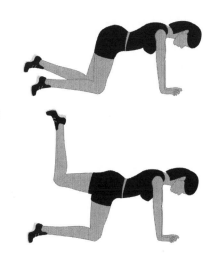

Crunches with Fitball

You may want to use a football, fitball, or bottle of water for this exercise. Try to lift shoulders off the floor as you reach forward then repeat.

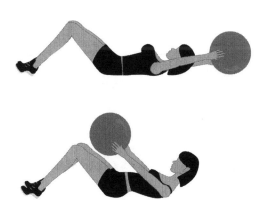

Circuit Workouts

In this section, there are 5 circuits for you to choose from.   Only attempt these when you have been regularly working out or you have been doing the exercises in the previous section and find your fitness level has improved.

Circuit 1

Toe taps

Front kicks

Twisting jump squats (Option is to take out the jump)

Bicycles

Clamshell

Flutter kicks

Knee plank

Duration: 30-45 seconds each exercise

Rest period between exercises: 15-30 seconds

Circuit sets: 3-5 (5 minutes rest between sets)

Healthy Black Life

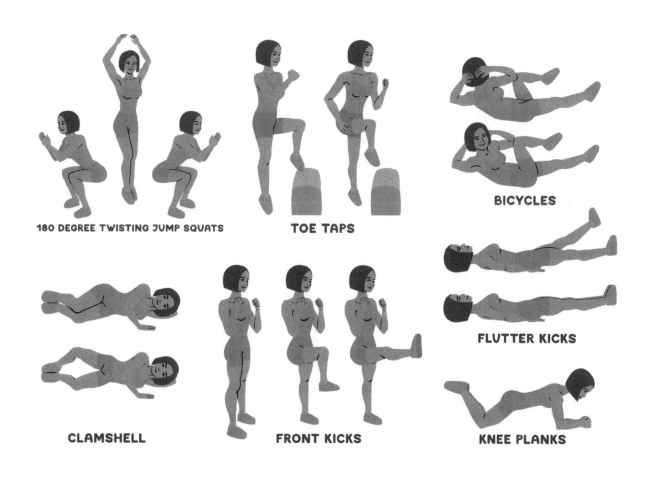

180 DEGREE TWISTING JUMP SQUATS

TOE TAPS

BICYCLES

CLAMSHELL

FRONT KICKS

FLUTTER KICKS

KNEE PLANKS

Circuit 2

Jumping jacks

Squats

Butt kicks

Wall sit

Lunges

Push ups

Sit ups

Crunches

Plank

Duration: 30-60 seconds

Rest period between exercises: 15-30 seconds

Circuit sets: 3-5 (5 minutes rest between sets)

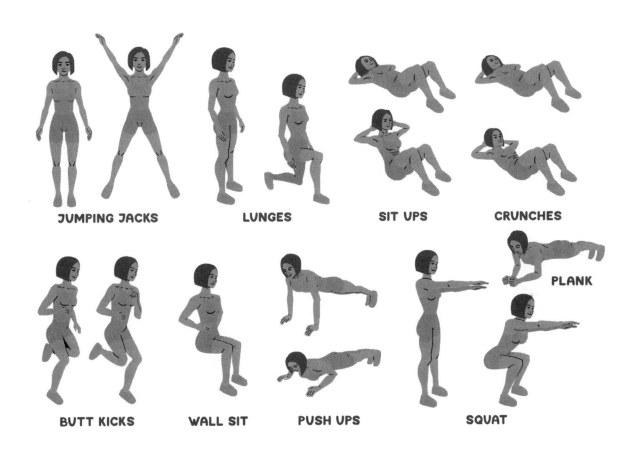

JUMPING JACKS   LUNGES   SIT UPS   CRUNCHES

BUTT KICKS   WALL SIT   PUSH UPS   PLANK   SQUAT

Let's Get Physical

Circuit 3

Squats

High knees

Chair dips (Use the sofa or a sturdy chair)

Low stance jacks

Punches

Mountain climbers

Leg raises

Knee pull-ins

Toe crunches

Duration of exercise: 30-60 seconds

Rest period between exercises: 15-30 seconds

Circuit sets: 3 -5 (5 minutes rest between sets)

Healthy Black Life

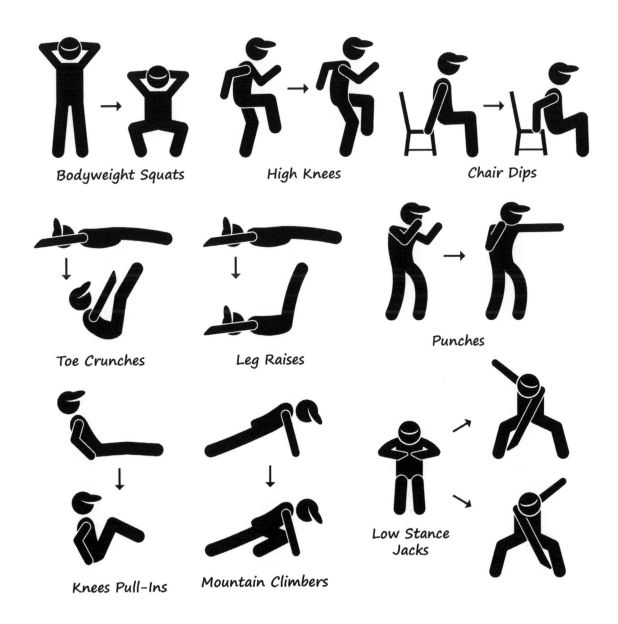

Bodyweight Squats

High Knees

Chair Dips

Toe Crunches

Leg Raises

Punches

Knees Pull-Ins

Mountain Climbers

Low Stance Jacks

Let's Get Physical

Core Exercise Circuit (For your back and abdominals)

Exercises for core strength will help improve and strengthen posture and tighten core muscles, toning your waist.

Choose 6-8 static core exercises

Duration: Hold the pose for 10-40 seconds - remember to breathe during the holding stage, as it's very easy to forget this.

You may find some of these exercises challenging, so stick with what you can do, and then as you become stronger, progress to the more challenging exercises.

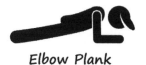

Elbow Plank

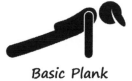

Basic Plank

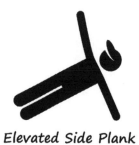

Elevated Side Plank

Elbow Plank (Knee)

Plank Leg Raise

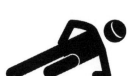

Ball Plank

Bent Knee Side Plank

Plank Arm Reach

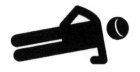

Side Plank

**Side Plank
Knee Tuck (1)**

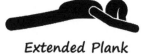

Ball Plank Reverse

Extended Plank

Side Plank Leg Lift

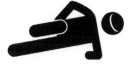

**Side Plank
Knee Tuck (2)**

Reverse Plank

Let's Get Physical

Dynamic Core Exercises

Choose 4-5 dynamic core exercises

Duration: 30-60 seconds

Rest period between exercises: 15-30 seconds

Circuit sets: 3-5 (5 minutes rest between sets)

Healthy Black Life

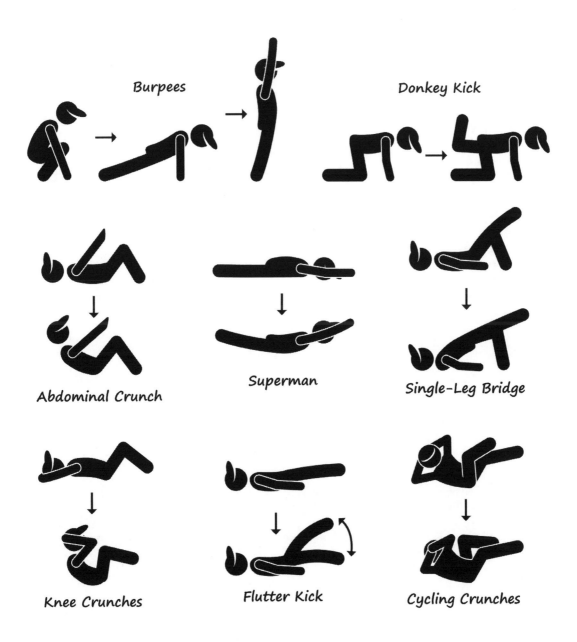

Burpees

Donkey Kick

Abdominal Crunch

Superman

Single-Leg Bridge

Knee Crunches

Flutter Kick

Cycling Crunches

Let's Get Physical

Chapter Nine

❖◆❖

Reducing Risk of Serious Disease & Easing Symptoms

Earlier in the book we touched on common diseases within the black community. This chapter offers further information and how to lower your risk of developing serious health concerns.

Remember, knowledge is power, so it is important to be equipped in order to make helpful and not harmful choices for your life. It may be useful to look back at Chapter 3 before you read on to familiarise yourself with what can cause disease.

Remember, knowledge is power, so it is important to be equipped in order to make helpful and not harmful choices for your life.

Hypertension (High Blood Pressure)

The most common way to find out if you have HBP is from a routine checkup at the doctor's office. Be aware that Hypertension over a prolonged period of time can lead to diseases such as:

- Stroke

- Heart Attack

- Kidney Disease

- Dementia (Due to lack of blood supply to the brain)

High Cholesterol

High Cholesterol can lead to:

- Stroke

- Cardiovascular Disease (Breathing Problems)

- Heart Disease

- Diabetes

Reduce the amount of salt in and on your food. Do this gradually so your tastebuds can adapt...

HBL Steps

- Go for a medical checkup with your GP

- Drink plenty of water to flush out excess Sodium (salt) and toxins in your blood vessels

- Reduce the amount of salt in and on your food. Do this gradually so your tastebuds can adapt to the flavour. Adding a little less salt each week is a good start.

- Take medication as prescribed

Healthy Black Life

- Move more
- Think about what you are eating and reduce fast food, fats, and sugar
- Reduce alcohol
- Stop smoking

The good news is that these two health concerns can be reversed by medication and a healthier diet and lifestyle. By looking after and loving yourself, you can tip the health scales in your favour, propelling you into a happier you and an increased quality of life. It's never too late to start making wiser lifestyle choices.

The good news is that these two health concerns can be reversed by medication and a healthier diet and lifestyle.

Type II Diabetes

Developing Type II diabetes increases the risk of other serious diseases and seems to be a real challenge for the Black and Asian communities.

Individuals with diabetes are at risk of developing the following diseases:

- Cardiovascular (Heart and Respiratory)
- Kidney
- Glaucoma (Eyes)
- Blindness

- Neuropathy (Nerve damage that affects the sensation in the lower limbs)
- Amputation
- Dementia
- Sexual Dysfunction
- Complications in Pregnancy
- Depression
- Reduced Life Expectancy

...Type II Diabetes can be kept under control and even reversed by physical exercise and making better dietary choices...

It is a medical fact that Type II diabetes can be kept under control and even reversed by physical exercise and making better dietary choices as discussed in previous chapters. You have the capacity to restore your health and well-being and increase your life expectancy. Over 400 million people around the world have been diagnosed with Type II diabetes, so this is a major worldwide problem. However, exact numbers may be higher as many individuals go undiagnosed, living with this condition not knowing they are diabetic.

Visit your GP as soon as possible if you experience the main symptoms of diabetes, which include:

- *feeling very thirsty*
- *peeing more frequently than usual, particularly at night*
- *feeling very tired*

- *weight loss and loss of muscle bulk*
- *itching around the penis or vagina, or frequent episodes of thrush*
- *cuts or wounds that heal slowly*
- *blurred vision[1]*

HBL Steps

If you have been diagnosed with diabetes:

- Drink water
- Eat healthier meals as described in this book
- Move more (i.e. Take up walking and fitness workouts)
- Reduce meal sizes
- Make a conscious effort to lose weight
- Limit your sugar and salt intake

Mental Health

Racial discrimination is a real and negative part of black history and life, and continues to exist everywhere. Experiencing discrimination can cause a degree of anxiety, consequently, impacting our attitude and mental health at any time in our life.
In years gone by, discrimination by the colour of our skin was more blatant, frequent,

---

1 https://www.nhs.uk/conditions/diabetes/

and acceptable. Whilst racism is less tolerated today, it still exists and can lead to depression and other mental health issues if experienced frequently. It's a fact that race and colour can put communities at a disadvantage in society, often resulting in living in lack and at the lower end of the socio-economic spectrum. Constantly being marginalised can create a very negative outlook in our thinking and our lives.

Whilst racism is less tolerated today, it still exists and can lead to depression and other mental health issues if experienced frequently.

We may start to believe these statements:

- Life will always be hard
- I will never have enough
- Situations will never be fair
- I will never be good enough
- There is no point trying
- There is no point dreaming or setting goals
- Nothing good will happen to me

It is not unusual to think this way when life is a struggle and you feel like a second-class citizen in the country you are living in. Because of this, you may look at life through the lens of a 'poverty mindset' which is the constant thought of living in lack, regardless of how much you actually have in your life. This thinking can influence how you approach situations in every area and can cause you to behave in certain ways. For instance, tightly holding on to material possessions and not throwing anything away and repeatedly

Healthy Black Life

talking about what you don't have. This mindset makes it difficult to be a dreamer or to set your sights on living a better life. To experience more in life, first you must see it through the eyes of your mind, your thinking, and believe 'good things can happen to me.'

To experience more in life, first you must see it through the eyes of your mind, your thinking, and believe 'good things can happen to me'.

Ask yourself the following questions and be totally honest with yourself so you can find out about your thinking habits.

- What do you find yourself thinking about when you wake up in the morning?
- Do you find yourself worrying about things too much? If so, what do you worry about?
- Do you imagine having more than what you have now?
- Are you suspicious of people?
- Do you get rid of old possessions or junk from time to time?
- Are you anxious about new things or situations?

To make changes in life, we first need to examine where we are right now. Pause and meditate on your answers to see whether your thinking has impaired your zest for life.

HBL Steps

If you experience regular anxiety or depression, it's important to seek help, whether that is through your faith group, community, or health service. Your mental health impacts every area of your life, so reach out and take those vital steps to help yourself. Our bodies need time to adjust to new habits and this is especially important for changing mindsets. So, do yourself a favour and think about what you are thinking about.

Please speak up and seek support if you are experiencing difficulty. Let's change our cultural habit and not suffer in silence.

Let's change our cultural habit and not suffer in silence.

Stroke

This information below was taken from the NHS website in the UK:

Ethnicity – if you're south Asian, African or Caribbean, your risk of stroke is higher, partly because rates of diabetes and high blood pressure are higher in these groups.[2]

Ischemic strokes
Ischemic strokes are the most common type of stroke. They happen when a blood clot blocks the flow of blood and oxygen to the brain.

These blood clots typically form in areas where the arteries have been narrowed or blocked over time by fatty deposits known as plaques. This process is known as atherosclerosis.

Your arteries may naturally become narrower as you age, but there are some things that dangerously speed up this process.

---

2 https://www.nhs.uk/conditions/stroke/causes/

Healthy Black Life

These include:

Smoking

High Blood Pressure (Hypertension)

Obesity

High Cholesterol Levels

Diabetes

Excessive Alcohol Intake[3]

The risks associated with a stroke resembles other health challenges discussed in this book. I hope you are starting to understand how one disease can manifest in to others especially if they are not addressed.

HBL Steps

- Stop smoking
- Reduce salt intake
- Reduce oil and sugar in diet
- Control alcohol consumption
- Exercise

---

3 https://www.nhs.uk/conditions/stroke/causes/

Lung Disease

During the Covid-19 pandemic, individuals with breathing issues were at higher risk of hospitalisation, because viral infections can severely affect the cardiovascular system.

Causes
- *Smoking*
- *Work related conditions such as fumes and dust*
- *Polluted air (indoors and outdoors)*

Still, too many of us smoke, even when we know the health implications, however this is more prevalent with men than women these days.[4]

Reports state that deprived areas with high populations and poorer living conditions are at a higher risk of developing breathing issues also. Therefore, it is safe to say that minority groups will inevitably be at risk of exposure.

Keeping your home clean is not just important if you are having guests coming over. It is also good for respiratory health. In this air polluted world we live in, it is important to keep our homes free from too many pollutants and keep the air circulating as much as possible, especially if you live in populated cities. In the UK, this is especially important in the winter months when we spend so much of our time indoors with the windows closed to keep warm. Drying our clothes indoors, cooking, and the steam from

4 https://www.statista.com/statistics/376602/cigarette-smoking-status-by-gender-in-england/

the bathroom can lead to high humidity in our homes. Our central heating can also be detrimental to our health by drying the air, as well as increasing black mould and damp spores. Homes can easily gather dust, which can increase dust mites in the atmosphere and affect our airways.

These events can increase breathing and lung problems, as well as contribute to adopting allergies and developing or worsening asthma.

...it is vital to address the air quality in your home, as it could be worsening your symptoms.

I recently found out via an Intolerance Test that I was 100% allergic to dust. Knowing this, I have increased dusting duties in my home, as I also suffer from hay-fever, and my symptoms are always worse when I'm home indoors.

So, if you are suffering with a lung disease like COPD (Chronic Obstructive Pulmonary Disease) or asthma, it is vital to address the air quality in your home, as it could be worsening your symptoms. When cleaning, try to use agents free of strong-smelling chemicals and bleach. There are many alternatives available in our supermarkets that are more friendly for our lungs and airways.

Not so long ago, I purchased a few small digital humidity gauges to check levels around the house. Some home weather stations can also display this information. Humidity levels above 55% are considered unhealthy, so when I notice the levels are high, I open a window to bring the humidity down and try to keep the house warm and not too hot in the winter.

Reducing Risk of Serious Disease & Easing Symptoms

HBL Steps

- Vacuum, mop, and dust home regularly.
- Use cleaning agents free of strong chemicals.
- Open windows all year round to improve circulation and reduce humidity.
- If possible, dry clothes in a tumble dryer or at the local laundrette instead of hanging clothes on a rack or over the radiators in the house, as the drying process increases humidity.
- Close kitchen and bathroom doors when cooking or having a shower/bath to keep the humidity confined to those rooms.
- Light exercise

Sickle Cell Disorder

Sickle cell disease is the name for a group of inherited health conditions that affect the red blood cells. The most serious type is called Sickle Cell Anaemia.

Sickle cell disease is particularly common in people with an African or Caribbean family background.

People with sickle cell disease produce unusually shaped red blood cells that can cause problems because they do not live as long as healthy blood cells and can block blood vessels.

Healthy Black Life

Sickle cell disease is a serious and lifelong health condition, although treatment can help manage many of the symptoms.

People with sickle cell disease need treatment throughout their lives. This is usually delivered by different health professionals in a specialist sickle cell centre.

It's also important for people with sickle cell disease to look after their own health using self care measures, such as by avoiding triggers and managing pain.[5]

Sickle cell is passed on genetically, but not all people who have the Sickle cell trait will suffer symptoms even though it can be passed down to offspring. The medical profession states that if an individual suffers from this disease, general health and well-being is important in reducing episodes/crises and symptoms.

...general health and well-being is important in reducing episodes/crises and symptoms.

HBL Steps

- Eat a balanced healthier diet
- Exercise
- Reduce stress

---

5 https://www.nhs.uk/conditions/sickle-cell-disease/

Uterine Fibroids

Why uterine fibroids are more prominent in people of colour is a mystery, but could our diet play a part in their development?

Rates of uterine fibroids are known to increase with age throughout the reproductive years, and it is well established that there is a higher prevalence among black women, who tend to have larger and more symptomatic fibroids than white women (1, 3, 7–10). A study of women undergoing hysterectomy for noncancerous conditions reported that 59% of the white women and 89% of black women had fibroids, with average age of diagnosis of 37.5 years in black women vs. 41.6 in white women (3). In the Nurses Health Study cohort of over 95,000 premenopausal females, the rate of new diagnoses of fibroids per year was reported as 12.8 per 1000 women-years, with the age-specific rate among black women peaking earlier than rates in other groups (8). However, only 5% of the study population was black (8). The Black Women's Health Study reported ultrasound and hysterectomy confirmed incidence rates as high as 29.7 per 1000 women-years, which translates to approximately 3% of premenopausal black women being diagnosed with fibroids yearly (10).[6]

---

6 https://www.ncbi.nlm.nih.gov/pmc/articles/PMC4465811/

Healthy Black Life

Uterine fibroids are non-malignant tumours that form in the uterus, but unfortunately, little is known about why they exist. The general consensus of the medical community is that they develop due to high levels of the hormone estrogen. As we age, this hormone can increase while our progesterone levels decrease (peri-menopause), resulting in a hormonal imbalance that causes fibroids to grow more rapidly.

Research suggests that certain foods and drink may contribute to their growth, implying our diet has an impact on their development.

Research suggests that certain foods and drink may contribute to their growth, implying our diet has an impact on their development. These tumours do not necessarily cause a serious health threat, however, depending on their size, they could potentially grow too large, making symptoms severe. It is not unusual for a woman to be unaware she has a fibroid, only to be discovered when suffering with menstrual issues or when pregnant. If the fibroid/s remain small once diagnosed, you may not experience any physical symptoms, therefore no further action will need to be taken.

I was diagnosed with a Uterine fibroid back in 2008, and after consultation, I decided to monitor the situation over the year. Over time, my symptoms worsened, so I returned to the doctor, who suggested I have a Merina coil fitted to help balance my hormones and reduce symptoms. My GP also mentioned that the fibroid could potentially shrink when I enter peri-menopause, however, he did not mention anything about changing my dietary habits.

Nothing improved over the next few years, and I was prescribed iron tablets as my symptoms were taking their toll on me. So, one day I decided to visit my doctor again to find out what was going on. After another scan, I was informed that the fibroid had grown to 11cm, and I was advised to have a Myomectomy to remove the mound, and after some thought, I nervously agreed to this procedure.

I reduced meat consumption, chose free range meats when possible, and reduced processed and starchy foods in my diet.

The week before surgery I went for my pre-op check, and within a few days the nurse called me to tell me they were cancelling surgery due to my blood count being far too low, probably due to anaemia. So, that was the end of that. I was never contacted again, so I chose to leave it, pray for healing, and research what I could do to help shrink it or reduce my symptoms. I tried a few different medications but I did not see much of a difference until I started to change my diet. I reduced meat consumption, chose free range meats when possible, and reduced processed and starchy foods in my diet. I also introduced raw and more green vegetables such as broccoli, spinach, and kale, as well as more colourful vegetables to increase macronutrients vital for good health.

After so many years of living with this benign tumour, I chose not to pursue surgery again as I was drawing closer to 50 years of age and the menopause. I am so thankful that my symptoms did, in fact, reduce considerably, and I no longer suffer like I did years ago. Hopefully, the fibroid has shrunk, however, I won't know until I return to my GP to schedule an appointment with the gynae for a scan.

Healthy Black Life

This is my story, and I'm sure everybody who has or had fibroids has a different experience, so I would suggest you visit your GP if you feel you have developed fibroids or if you are having major menstrual issues.

What I believe helped reduce my symptoms were:

- Increasing my vegetable intake and eating raw vegetables
- Reduction of meat
- Eating more organic fresh produce
- My age (menopausal)

Chapter 10

— ◆●◆ —

One Step at a Time to a Healthy Black Life
-
An Epilogue

I truly hope that this book has informed, encouraged, and inspired you to really take a good look at your life and take small steps to increase your health, and keep up with your family and children's children. My intention is for you to use this book as a reference to support

...re-read sections depending on where you are on your health journey.

your everyday life and to re-read sections depending on where you are on your health journey.

I thoroughly enjoy helping people increase their fitness, lose weight, and reach their goals. There are generally highs and lows along the way and this is normal, especially when you are trying to change lifelong habits and manage your emotions. But, the joy of those who improve their health reminds me of how much pleasure I get from seeing lives positively change. I have an increasing desire to see more of the black community taking steps to improve their health (especially those over the age of 35) since the rise of the Covid-19 pandemic. I have encountered so many who struggle to improve their health, so I wrote this book in order to meet a need in our community that weighs heavy on my heart, and I also hope that we start to reverse the current trend of poor health. Writing a book enables me to reach more people and share my God given knowledge and expertise as a Fitness Trainer and Health Coach across the globe.

I spent my younger years watching sport on TV trying to image myself as a top athlete and eventually became a pretty good sprinter back in the day. There was so much sport on television, I was drawn towards being fit and achieving sporting success. I was on most of the sports teams at school and even won 1987 Sportsperson of the year at my school leaving ceremony. I truly believe watching sport had a huge impact on my life and played a part in bringing me to where I am today. However, over the past few decades it saddened me to see that many sports have disappeared from terrestrial (free) TV, and now to watch these great sportsmen and women reaching great heights in their career, we have to pay extra for it via the cable and satellite networks. Limiting access purely for profit reduces the opportunity to encourage and nurture the next generation to dream of becoming athletes or to just encourage them to be more active. The explosion of technology and social media has made it even more difficult to persuade the younger generation to value movement and their health. I still love to watch sport; it energizes me, even the fishing programmes, ask my hubby!

Healthy Black Life

As I mentioned at the beginning of the book, my father passed away at the age of 53 from heart disease, after having a previous bypass operation in his 40s. Back then, I did not understand the extent of his health issues, as I very rarely saw him unwell. I was twenty years old when I visited my father for the last time in St Thomas' Hospital London. The nurse had told him his daughter was visiting him that day, and when I walked into the ward, he looked surprised to see me; I think he was expecting my older sister instead. I will never forget the last chat we had together, and for the first time, I felt like we had a grown-up conversation. We spoke about healthier eating and his lifestyle, and I advised him about certain foods he needed to reduce and those he needed to include in his diet. We had never spoken like that before (he had left the family home around eight years prior and had remarried). He passed away not too long after my hospital visit and at the wake after his funeral, his wife came over to me and said she had a cupboard full of sardines that my father had told her to buy because I had said they were good for his health. At that moment, amongst the sorrow I was feeling, it brought a smile to my face and warmth to my heart. He had acted on my advice and was determined to take steps to improve his health. But unfortunately, it was too late!

I will never forget the last chat we had together, and for the first time, I felt like we had a grown-up conversation.

Share your efforts and achievements with one another and encourage each other every step of the way.

While writing this book, tragedy hit us hard when my younger brother Jimmy passed away suddenly attributed to a heart condition, just before his 50th birthday. This was devastating for our family and his closest friends. To be honest, I found it difficult to continue to write this book, as the subject was so close to home, and thinking about the book reminded me of Jim, our grief, and our shattered hearts. A few months on, after leaning on God, He gave me the strength and courage to finish this book, with an increased desire to help those who want to improve their health.

Share your efforts and achievements with one another and encourage each other every step of the way. Look after your body, mind, and spirit, and live a blessed Healthy Black Life!

Paula Watson Gardner

In Loving Memory

of

James Sylvester Watson